Quick and easy renal diet recipes

Cookbook with 50 Flavorful Recipes for all stages of kidney disease. Especially designed for beginners

ALEXANDRA DAVID

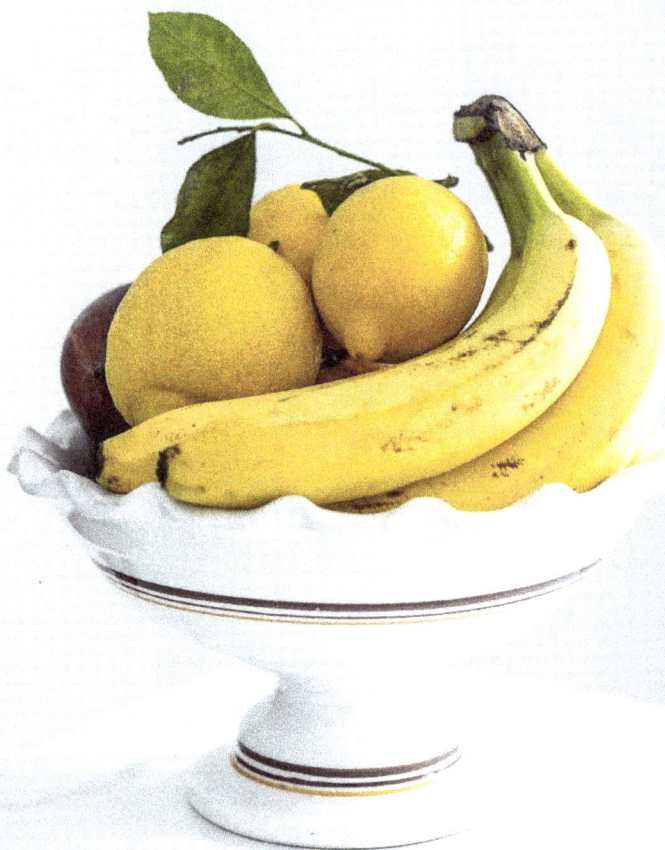

TABLE OF CONTENTS

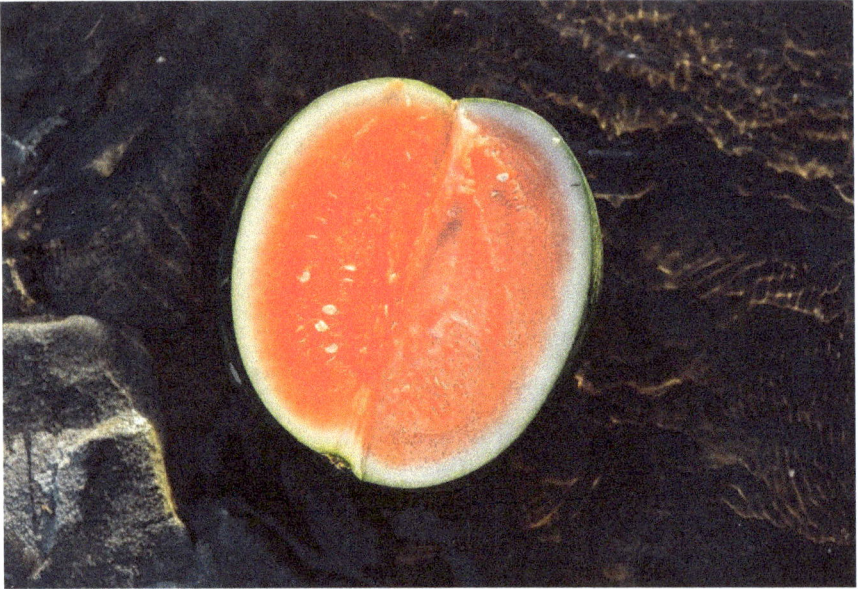

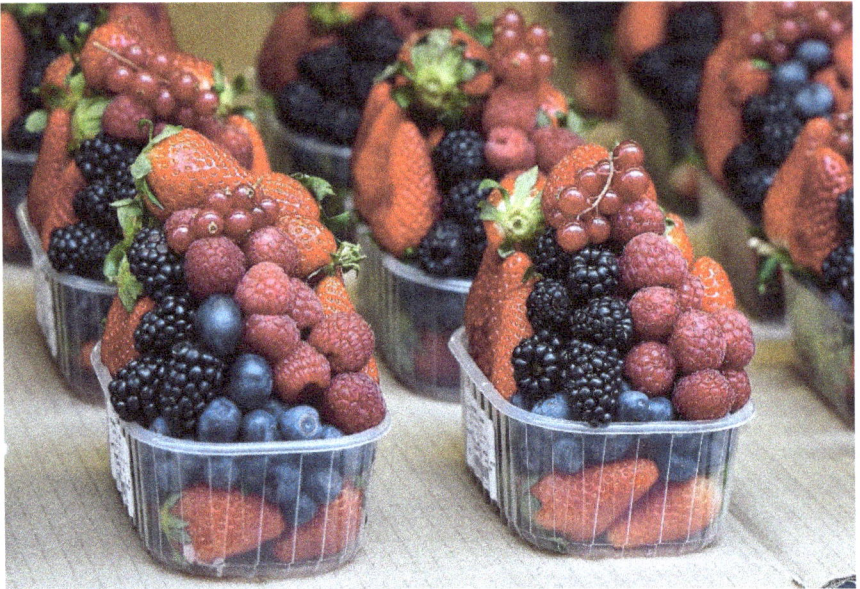

Introduction

Kidney disease is a common condition in which the filtering and excretory function of the kidney is increasingly lost. Several underlying diseases can be the cause; first and foremost are years of diabetes and hypertension. Early diagnosis and treatment can, in many cases, slow the progression of the disease to a point where the end-stage with dialysis or kidney transplantation does not occur.

The most effective remedy for chronic renal failure is the prevention of widespread diabetes and hypertension diseases.

The kidneys are two bean-shaped organs 10-12 cm in length, which lie on either side of the spine below the diaphragm. They contain a complex filter system that removes toxic substances and excess water from the blood while at the same time retaining required substances.. Depending on the requirements of the body, the amount, concentration, and composition of the urine change.

Other tasks of the kidney are the influence on the blood pressure and the production of important hormones for blood formation and calcium metabolism.

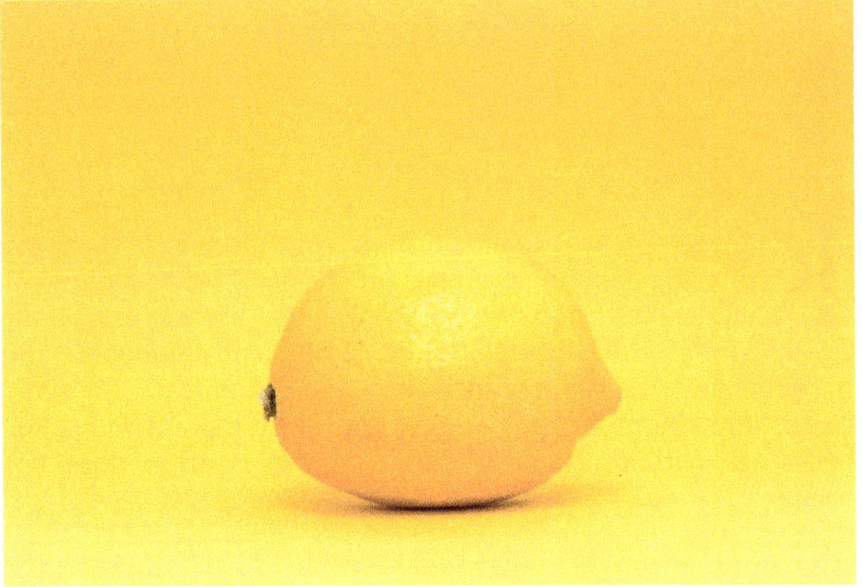

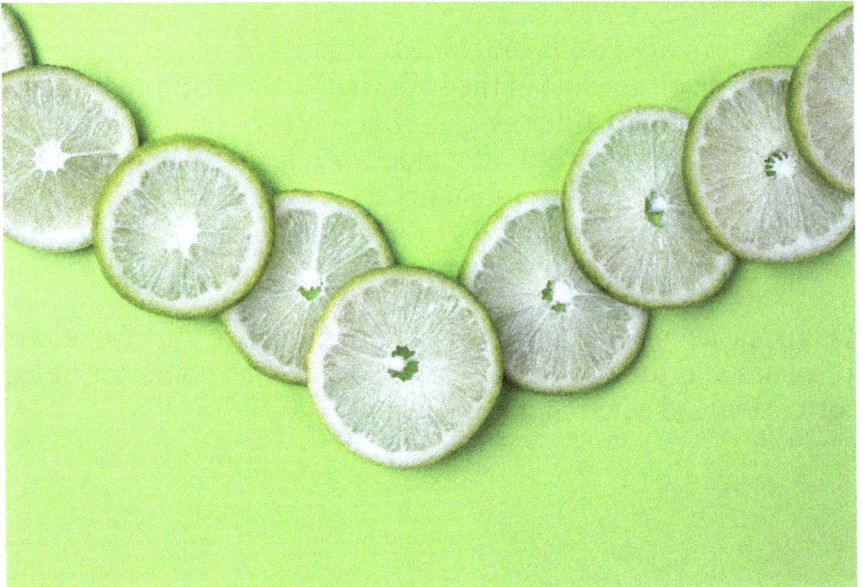

CHAPTER 1:

Renal Diet

A renal diet means eating with an emphasis on promoting the kidney's health. It is recommended for anyone who is suffering from renal disease to reduce the progression and complications of that disease, such as electrolyte imbalance, anemia, heart disease, ETC. It includes restrictions on certain micronutrients such as sodium, potassium, phosphorus, proteins, and input of fluids. A person may need to limit their consumption of vegetables, fruits, grains, and red meat. There is great importance given to what type of protein should be eaten. Different people experience different types of renal diseases, and according to their condition, they'll need to change their diet. Some people only limit salt in their diet, and some people need to focus more on their potassium intake. You may need to discuss this with a doctor or a qualified dietitian so you can get the best possible outcome from the diet.

Micronutrients for Renal Diet

There are many nutrients that a person suffering from renal disease must monitor. Some of them are:

S

Potassium

This is also a very important nutrient needed for the function of the heart. It is found in many foods. It is also important for the healthy function of muscles as well. Potassium increases when kidneys do not function properly, and when this happens, it is called hyperkalemia. This can cause a series of heart problems such as arrhythmias, muscle degeneration, cardiac attack and paralysis. You can decrease your potassium intake by:

- Reading packaging labels for potassium levels

- Eating fresh vegetables and fruits

- Avoiding foods with a high level of potassium

- Keeping track of how much potassium you are eating in a day.

Phosphorus

This is also an important micronutrient for the body's healthy functions. It is important for bone development, growth of certain organs, and connective tissues. If the kidneys are not working properly, then phosphorus will accumulate inside the body. Phosphorus takes out the calcium from the bones into the blood, making the bones weaker and increasing the level of calcium in the blood dangerously.

To keep track of phosphorus, you can:

- Read the packaging labels for levels of phosphorus

- Avoid eating foods with a high level of phosphorus

- Eat high quality and low-fat meat

- Eat fresh fruits and vegetables.

Proteins

High levels of protein and amino acids in the blood occur when the kidneys cannot filter the excess protein properly out of the body. The broken-down proteins and their waste products circulate the body's system, causing a lot of problems. It damages the structures of the kidneys as well.

The amount of protein a person needs to consume is tricky because it depends upon the individual's condition. Overall, there is an emphasis on eating high-quality protein and reducing the amount of red meat. For complete guidance, consult a doctor or dietitian.

Water intake can be a problem when the kidneys are not functioning properly. Excess water inside the body cannot be filtered out without the help of dialysis in extreme cases.

To reduce the load on the kidneys, drink as low amounts of fluid as possible. Excess fluid can cause damage to other organs, such as the heart and lungs, by putting more pressure on them.

You can keep track of your fluid intake by:

• Avoiding salty and spicy foods

• Taking medicine with sips of water

• Keeping a record of fluid intake along with your food in a journal

• Avoiding salty condiments, such as soy sauce

• Drinking cold fluids

• Following instructions from professionals on what to drink and what not to drink.

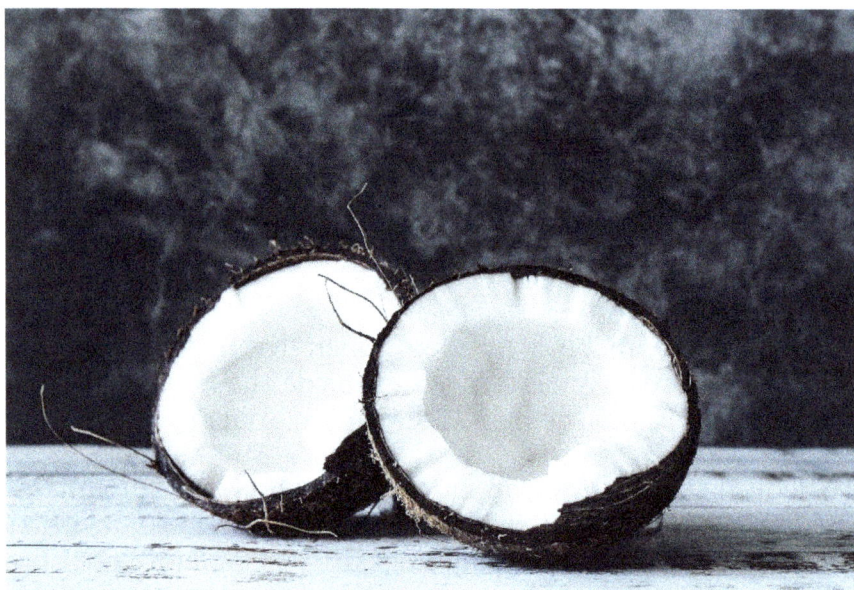

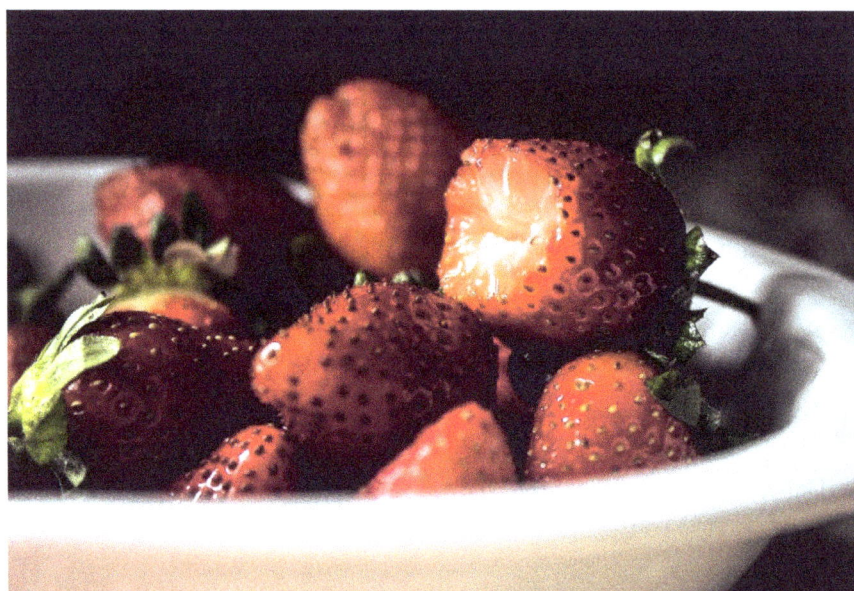

CHAPTER 2:

What You Can Eat and What You Can Avoid in Renal Diet

Food to Eat

The renal diet aims to cut down the amount of waste in the blood. When people have kidney dysfunction, the kidneys are unable to remove and filter waste properly. When waste is left in the blood, it can affect the electrolyte levels of the patient. With a kidney diet, kidney function is promoted, and the progression of complete kidney failure is slowed down.

The renal diet follows a low intake of protein, phosphorus, and sodium. It is necessary to consume high-quality protein and limit some fluids. For some people, it is important to limit calcium and potassium.

Promoting a renal diet, here are the substances which are critical to be monitored:

Potassium and Its Role in the Body

The main function of potassium is keeping muscles working correctly and the heartbeat regular. This mineral is responsible for maintaining electrolyte and fluid balance in the bloodstream. The kidneys regulate the proper amount of potassium in the body, expelling excess amounts in the urine.

Monitoring potassium intake:

- Limit high potassium food

- Select only fresh fruits and veggies

- Limit dairy products and milk to 8 oz. per day

- Avoid potassium chloride

- Read labels on packaged foods

- Avoid seasonings and salt substitutes with potassium.

Foods to eat with lower potassium:

- Fruits: watermelon, tangerines, pineapple, plums, peaches, pears, papayas, mangoes, lemons and limes, honeydew, grapefruit/grapefruit juice, grapes/grape juice, clementine/Satsuma, cranberry juice, berries, and apples/ applesauce, apple juice

- Veggies: summer squash (cooked), okra, mushrooms (fresh), lettuce, kale, green beans, eggplant, cucumber, corn, onions (raw), celery, cauliflower, carrots, cabbage, broccoli (fresh), bamboo shoots (canned), and bell peppers

- Plain Turkish delights, marshmallows and jellies, boiled fruit sweets, and peppermints

- Shortbread, ginger nut biscuits, plain digestives

- Plain flapjacks and cereal bars

- Plain sponge cakes like Madeira cake, lemon sponge, jam sponge

- Corn-based and wheat crisps

- Whole grain crisp breads and crackers

- Protein and other foods (bread (not whole grain), pasta, noodles, rice, eggs, canned tuna, turkey (white meat), and chicken (white meat).

Phosphorus and Its Role in the Body

This mineral is essential in bone development and maintenance. Phosphorus helps in the development of connective organs and tissue and assists in muscle movement. Extra phosphorus is possible to be removed by healthy kidneys. However, it is impossible with kidney dysfunction. High levels of phosphorus make bones weak by pulling calcium out of your bones. It might lead to dangerous calcium deposits in the heart, eyes, lungs, and blood vessels.

Monitoring phosphorus intake:

- Pay attention to serving size

- Eat fresh fruits and veggies

- Eat smaller portions of foods that are rich in protein

- Avoid packaged foods

- Keep a food journal.

Foods to eat with low phosphorus level:

- Grapes, apples

- Lettuce, leeks

- Carbohydrates (white rice, corn, and rice cereal, popcorn, pasta, crackers, —not wheat—and white bread)

- Meat (sausage, fresh meat).

Protein

Damaged kidneys are unable to remove protein waste, so they accumulate in the blood. The amount of protein to consume differs depending on the stage of CKD. Protein is critical for tissue maintenance, and it is necessary to eat the proper amount of it according to the particular stage of kidneys disease. Sources of protein for vegetarians:

- Vegans (allowing only plant-based foods): Wheat protein and whole grains, nut butter, soy protein, yogurt or soy milk, cooked no salt added canned and dried beans and peas, unsalted nuts.

- Lacto vegetarians (allowing dairy products, milk, and plant-based foods): reduced-sodium or low-sodium cottage cheese.

- Lacto-ovo vegetarians (allowing eggs, dairy products, milk, and plant-based foods): eggs.

Food to Avoid

Food with High Sodium Content:

- Onion salt, marinades, garlic salt, teriyaki sauce, and table salt Pepperoni, bacon, ham, lunch meat, hot dogs, sausage, processed meats

- Ramen noodles, canned produce, and canned soups

- Marinara sauce, gravy, salad dressings, soy sauce, BBQ sauce, and ketchup Chex Mix, salted nuts, Cheetos, crackers, and potato chips

- Fast food.

Food with a High Potassium Level:

- Fruits: dried fruit, oranges/orange juice, prunes/prune juice, kiwi, nectarines, dates, cantaloupe, bananas, black currants, damsons, cherries, grapes, and apricots.

- Vegetables: tomatoes/tomato sauce/tomato juice, sweet potatoes, beans, lentils, split peas, spinach (cooked), pumpkin, potatoes, mushrooms (cooked), chile peppers, chard, Brussels sprouts (cooked), broccoli (cooked), baked beans, avocado, butternut squash, and acorn squash.

- Protein and other foods: peanut butter, molasses, granola, chocolate, bran, sardines, fish, bacon, ham, nuts and seeds, yogurt, milkshakes, and milk.

- Coconut-based snacks, nut-based snacks, fudge, and toffee.

- Cakes containing marzipan.

- Potato crisps.

Foods with High Phosphorus:

- Dairy products: pudding, ice cream, yogurt, cottage cheese, cheese, and milk.

- Nuts and seeds: sunflower seeds, pumpkin seeds, pecans, peanut butter, pistachios, cashews, and almonds. Dried beans and peas: soybeans, split peas, refried beans, pinto beans, lentils, kidney beans, garbanzo beans, black beans, and baked beans.

- Meat: veal, turkey, liver, lamb, beef, bacon, fish, and seafood.

- Carbohydrates: whole grain products, oatmeal, and bran cereals.

CHAPTER 3:

Renal Diet and Its Benefits

If you have been diagnosed with kidney dysfunction, a proper diet is necessary for controlling the amount of toxic waste in the bloodstream. When toxic waste piles up in the system along with increased fluid, chronic inflammation occurs, and we have a much higher chance of developing cardiovascular, bone, metabolic, or other health issues.

The above-mentioned benefits are noticeable once the patient follows the diet for at least a month and then continuing it for longer periods to avoid the stage where dialysis is needed. The strictness of the diet depends on the current stage of renal/kidney disease. If, for example, you are in the 3rd or 4th stage, you should follow a stricter diet and be attentive to the food, which is allowed or prohibited.

These exact foods and nutrients that you should take when following a renal diet will be given to you in the following sections, and so keep on reading.

Explanation of Key Diet Words

The following nutrients play a major role in a renal diet as some have the ability to improve the condition while others can make it worse. Essentially, the renal diet is based on low consumption of certain nutrients like potassium and phosphorus simply because it promotes fluid buildup within the system of a kidney patient. Here is a brief explanation of the function of each nutrient and its role in a renal diet.

Potassium

Potassium is a mineral that naturally occurs in certain foods and plays a role in regulating heart rhythm and muscle movement. It is also needed for keeping fluid and electrolyte balance at normal levels. Our kidneys keep only the right levels of potassium in our system, and when it is excess, they expel it via the urine.

The problem is, once kidneys can't function properly, all this excess potassium can't be expelled out and spikes up, causing symptoms like muscle and bone weakness, abnormal heartbeat, and heart failure in extreme cases.

Thus, a diet low in potassium is recommended to prevent buildup and avoid such negative side effects.

Sodium

Sodium is a trace mineral that is found in most foods that we eat today, and it is the key component of salt, which is actually a sodium compound mixed with chloride. Most food that we consume and especially processed food is highly loaded with salt; however, we may be eating sodium in other forms too, e.g., fish. The key role of sodium is to regulate blood pressure, help regulate nerve function, and maintain the balance of acids in the blood. However, when sodium is excessively high, and the kidneys can expel it, it can lead to the following symptoms: an elevated feeling of thirst, swelling of hands, feet, and the face elevated blood pressure, and problems with breathing.

This is why it is suggested to keep sodium intake low to avoid the above.

Phosphorus

Phosphorus is an essential mineral that is responsible for the development and regeneration of our bones. Phosphorus also plays a key role in the growth of connective tissue e.g. muscles and the regulation of muscle motions. When the food we take contains phosphorus, it gets absorbed by the intestines and then gets deposited in our bones.

However, when kidneys are damaged or dysfunctioning, the excess phosphorus can't be expelled through our systems and causes problems such as: extracting calcium out of the bones/making them weaker, and leading to excess calcium in the bloodstream, which interferes with blood vessels, heart, eye, and lung function.

Protein

Protein is a nutritional compound that consists of amino acids, which play a key role in various system functions like cell communication, oxygen supply, and cellular metabolism. They are also a part of a healthy immune system.

Normally, protein is not an issue for our kidneys. When protein is metabolized, waste by-products are also created and are filtered through the kidneys. This waste, along with extrarenal proteins after will be expelled through urine.

However, when kidneys are unable to filter out excess protein, it gets accumulated in the blood and cause problems.

This doesn't mean that renal disease patients should avoid protein totally as it is still necessary for some metabolic functions, as long as it's taken in moderate amounts and based on the stage of renal disease.

Carbs

Carbs act as a key source of fuel for our bodies. The consumption of carbs is turned into glucose in our system, which is a primary source of energy.

Carbs are ok to be eaten in moderation by kidney patients, and the daily recommended allowance is up to 150 grams/day. However, patients that also suffer from diabetes (besides renal disease) should control their carb consumption to avoid any sudden spikes in their blood glucose.

Fats

Being in balanced amounts, fats in our bodies act as an energy source, aid in the release of hormones, and help regulate blood pressure. They also carry some vitamins that are fat-soluble such as A, D, E, and K, which are also very important for our systems. Not all fats are created equal though some are good for our health, and some are bad. Bad fats are saturated, like trans fats found in processed meat, dairy, and other products. They are also found in margarine and vegetable fat shortening. Fats, in general, don't pose a risk for renal disease patients, however, it is suggested to limit the consumption of saturated and trans fats to avoid any cardiovascular problems, e.g., elevated blood pressure and clogging of the arteries.

Dietary fiber

Dietary fiber is a compound that can't be digested on its own by enzymes and acids in our stomach and intestines but is needed for the system to aid in the digestion of our food and encourage bowel movements. They generally promote bowel regularity and decrease the likelihood of developing constipation inside the colon. Dietary fiber is typically found in fruits, vegetables, seeds, and whole grains. In patients with renal disease, dietary fiber is ok up to 28 grams/day as long as these plant foods don't contain high amounts of phosphorus or potassium.

Vitamins

According to medical and dietary guidelines, our bodies need close to 13 vitamins to functions. Vitamins play a key role in metabolic functions and the normal functioning of our cardiovascular, digestive, nervous system, and immune systems. The adoption of a nutritionally dense and balanced diet is necessary for getting all the vitamins our system needs. However, due to some diet restrictions e.g., sodium, many renal patients are in need of water-soluble vitamins like B-complex (B1, B2, B6, B12, folic acid, biotin) and small amounts of Vitamin C.

Minerals

Minerals are needed for our system to maintain healthy connective tissue e.g., bones, muscles, and skin, and facilitate the normal function of our hearts and central nervous systems.

Other trace minerals are perfectly fine when following a renal diet: iron, copper, zinc, and selenium. A lack of these can lead to increased oxidative stress, and thus, it is important to take sufficient amounts through diet or supplementation.

Fluids

However, in patients with renal dysfunction, fluids can quickly build-up to the point of placing pressure on vital organs like the lungs and heart and becoming dangerous. This is why many physicians advise their kidney patients to limit the consumption of fluids, especially during the last stages of the disorder.

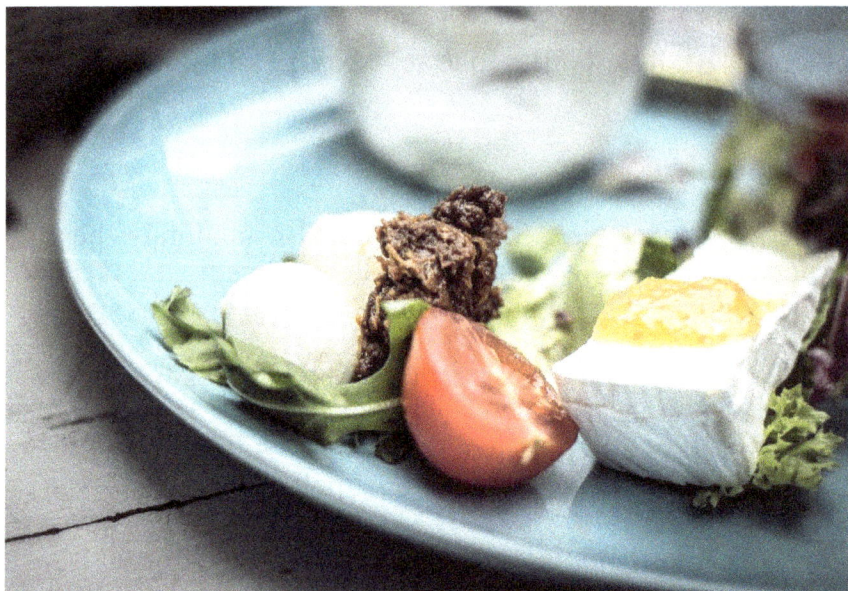

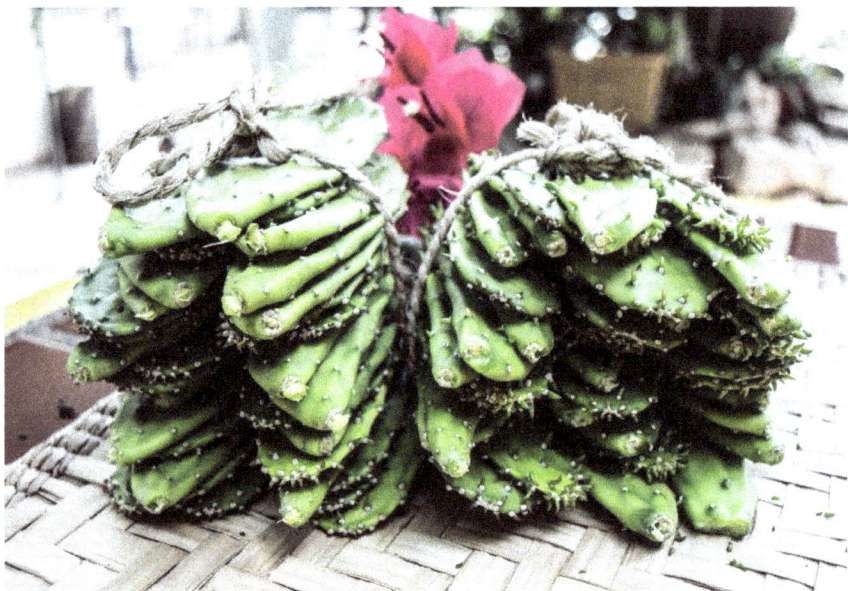

CHAPTER 4:

30 Day Meal Plan

Diets are easier when you have a definitive meal plan in your hands. This 30-day meal plan specifically for the renal diet, will help you enjoy all the flavors and nutrients found in this cookbook easily.

MEAL PLAN	BREAKFAST	LUNCH	DINNER		SNACK
Day 1	Apple Onion Omelet	Chicken Wild Rice Soup	Braised Beef Brisket		Chicken Pepper Bacon Wraps
Day 2	Apple Fritter Rings	Chicken Noodle Soup	California Pork Chops		Chicken Pepper Bacon Wraps
Day 3	Apple Cinnamon Maple Granola	Cucumber Soup	Beef Chorizo		Buffalo Chicken Dip
Day 4	Asparagus and Cheese Crepe Rolls with Parsley	Squash and Turmeric Soup	Pork Fajitas		Shrimp Spread with Crackers

Day 5	Acai Berry Smoothie Bowl	Wild Rice Asparagus Soup	Caribbean Turkey Curry		Garlic Oyster Crackers
Day 6	Baked Egg Cups	Nutmeg Chicken Soup	Chicken with Rosemary-Garlic Sauce		Vanilla Delight
Day 7	Belgian Waffles	Hungarian Cherry Soup	Chicken Fajitas		Sweet and Spicy Tortilla Chips
Day 8	Clam Omelet	Italian Wedding Soup	Chicken with Rosemary-Garlic Sauce		Turnip Chips
Day 9	Leek Cauliflower Tortilla	Old Fashioned Salmon Soup	Chicken Paprika		Sweet Savory Meatballs
Day 10	Cottage Cheese Sour Cream Pancakes	Oxtail Soup	Grilled Chicken Masala		Apple Cranberry Slaw
Day 11	Apple Onion Omelet	Old Fashioned Salmon Soup	Chicken with Rosemary-Garlic Sauce		Asian Cabbage Slaw
Day 12	Apple Fritter Rings	Oxtail Soup	Caribbean Turkey Curry		Autumn Orzo Salad

Day 13	Acai Berry Smoothie Bowl	Hungarian Cherry Soup	Chicken Fajitas		Basil-Lime Pineapple Salad
Day 14	Asparagus and Cheese Crepe Rolls with Parsley	Italian Wedding Soup	Chicken with Rosemary-Garlic Sauce		Creamy Cucumber Salad
Day 15	Apple Cinnamon Maple Granola	Nutmeg Chicken Soup	Chicken Paprika		Basil-Lime Pineapple Salad
Day 16	Baked Egg Cups	Squash and Turmeric Soup	Grilled Chicken Masala		Tortilla Wraps
Day 17	Belgian Waffles	Simple Soup	Baked Pork Chops		Garden Vegetable Salad
Day 18	Clam Omelet	Cucumber Soup	Braised Beef Brisket		Green Pepper Slaw
Day 19	Confetti Omelet	Chicken Noodle Soup	California Pork Chops		Cranberry Cream Salad
Day 20	Apple Onion Omelet	Chicken Wild Rice Soup	Baked Pork Chops		Creamy Cucumber Salad
Day 21	Cottage Cheese Sour Cream Pancakes	Squash and Turmeric Soup	Grilled Salmon		Cucumber-Carrot Salad

Day 22	Macaroni and Cheese	Simple Soup	Cabbage Bake		Mushroom Stuffing Balls
Day 23	Onion Quiche	Crispy Fish Fillets	Chicken Cabbage Soup		Garlic, Mint Deviled Eggs
Day 24	Zucchini with Egg	Turkey and Vegetable Bake	Lemon Dijon Chicken		Japanese Deviled Eggs
Day 25	Spanish Omelette with Zucchini	White Fish Soup	Grilled Lamb Steaks with Rosemary		Garlic, Mint Deviled Eggs
Day 26	Cheesesteak Quiche	Almond Lemon Turkey	Lamb Keema		Balsamic Mushrooms
Day 27	Soy Milk Pancakes	Fruity Chicken Salad	Spicy Chicken Breasts		Maple Summer Squash Chips
Day 28	Pumpkin Spiced Muffin	French Crepes	Rosemary Shrimp		Herbed Raspberries Salsa
Day 29	Spaghetti-Parsley Frittata	Citrus Baked Fish	Stir-Fry Vegetables		Zesty Duck Wings
Day 30	Salmon Omelette	Grilled Lamb Chops with Fresh	Lemon-Pepper Salmon with Couscous		Pita Chips

CHAPTER 5:

Breakfast Recipes

1. Egg Cups

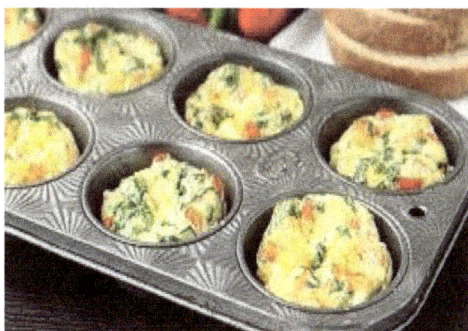

Preparation time: 10 minutes

Cooking time: 30 minutes

Servings: 12

Ingredients:

- ¼ cup shiitake mushrooms—diced

- 1/3 cup bell peppers—diced

- 1/3 cup onion—diced

- 12 eggs

- ½ teaspoon oregano—dried or fresh.

Directions:

As you are cutting and washing vegetables and mushrooms, make sure that your oven is preheated to 350 degrees F° and that your baking dish is ready. You can place a tin foil over the baking dish and arrange 12 muffin cups.

The next step is to take a bowl and beat the eggs, and add oregano. Let the eggs rest while you take care of the veggies and mushrooms. Take a frying pan or any kind of cooking dish, add some olive oil, not more than a tablespoon, and sauté the onion. After several minutes of sautéing and stirring, add peppers and mushrooms to the pan and sauté some more until the veggies are mildly softened, and the onion is slightly browned. Add the veggie mixture to the bowl with eggs, combine it all well with a spoon then fill muffin cups with the mixture you have prepared. Place the baking dish into the oven and bake for 25 minutes.

Nutrition:

- Potassium: 90mg

- Sodium: 70mg

- Phosphorus: 100mg

- Calories: 80.

2. Breakfast Casserole

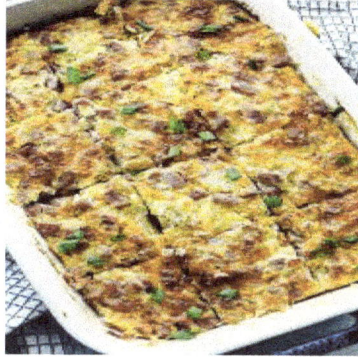

Preparation time: 10 minutes

Cooking time: 60 minutes

Servings: 8

Ingredients:

- 200 grams of lean ground beef—fresh and grass-fed if possible

- ½ cup cream cheese

- 4 slices of bread white, cut in cubes

- 5 eggs

- 1 teaspoon of mustard—dry

- ½ teaspoon garlic powder with no added sodium.

Directions:

Preheat your oven to 350 degrees F as you are preparing ingredients for the breakfast casserole. Cube bread sliced and place it aside while you are taking care of the ground beef. As you prepare the beef, add a tablespoon of olive oil to the skillet and add the beef. Cook the beef with occasional stirring as you are breaking the meat parts to bits. Once the meat is browned, set aside and add garlic powder, stirring it well to combine. Beat the five eggs in a bowl, then combine all ingredients in the egg bowl, and mix to get a homogenous mass out of the egg mixture. Pour the mixture into the mildly greased baking dish and place it in the oven. Bake for 50 minutes or until ready.

Nutrition:

- Potassium: 176mg

- Sodium: 201mg

- Phosphorus: 119mg

- Calories: 220.

3. Grilled Veggie and Cheese Bagel

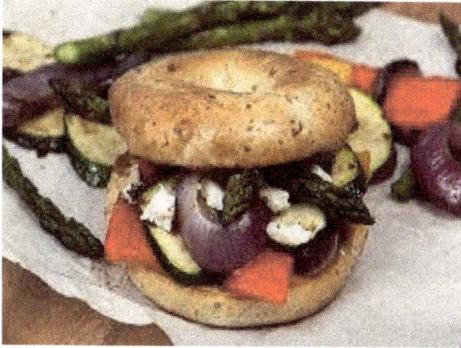

Preparation time: 10 minutes

Cooking time: 5 minutes

Servings: 1

Ingredients:

- 1 white flour bagel—sliced in half

- ½ cup arugula

- ½ cup low-sodium cheese or cream cheese (lower potassium, higher sodium)

- ¼ red onion—finely sliced

- 2 slices eggplant—roasted or grilled

- ½ teaspoon lemon pepper.

Directions:

First, you need to deal with preparing veggies and slicing, and once the preparation is finished, grill 2 slices of eggplant with some lemon pepper spread over the slices.

Baking the eggplant slices would be another option in case you don't have an option to grill the slices.

 You may roast the eggplant by placing it on a tin foil or a baking paper set on a baking dish in a preheated oven for 5 minutes each side of the slices.

Once the eggplant is grilled, toast the bagel sliced in two as for making a sandwich the same way the eggplant was grilled, but reduced to grilling each side 2 minutes or less.

Spread some cheese on the bagel, add the eggplant slices and the rest of the ingredients.

Seal the bagel with the top part, and you have a great start to the day.

Nutrition:

- Potassium: 112mg

- Sodium: 186mg

- Phosphorus: 50mg

- Calories: 114.

4. Cauliflower Tortilla

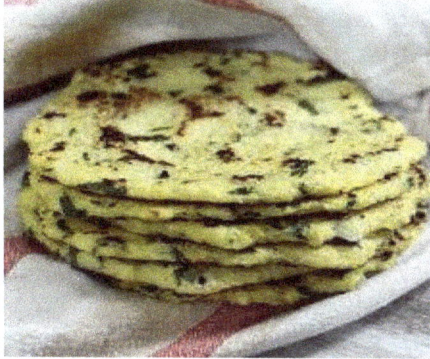

Preparation time: 10 minutes

Cooking time: 20 minutes

Servings: 4

Ingredients:

- 4 cups cauliflower

- 1 cup onion—chopped

- 2 garlic cloves—minced

- 1 cup egg substitute—liquefied

- ¼ teaspoon nutmeg

- 1 tablespoon parsley—fresh, chopped

- ½ teaspoon allspice.

Direction:

Prepare the cauliflower by cutting it into small cubes, then place the cauliflower bits in a bowl with a tablespoon of water and microwave it for 5 minutes until the cauliflower is crisped.

While you are waiting for the cauliflower bits to get ready in the microwave, you may start preparing the onion. Sauté chopped onions with 2 tablespoons of olive oil until browned, which should take around 5 minutes, add garlic, nutmeg, and allspice to the pan. Stir in and cook for another 1 to 2 minutes, then add the cauliflower and egg substitute. Stir in all ingredients to combine the mixture, then seal the pan and lower the heat. Cook for another 10 to 15 minutes, until cauliflower tortilla is browned. Serve by slicing the tortilla into 4 pieces.

Nutrition:

- Potassium: 272mg

- Sodium: 148mg

- Phosphorus: 78mg

- Calories: 102.

5. Eggs Benedict

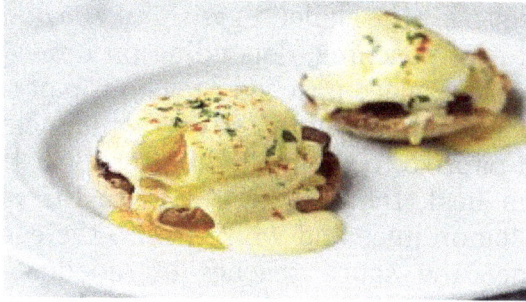

Preparation time: 10 minutes

Cooking time: 15 minutes

Servings: 4

Ingredients:

- 2 pieces of toasted bread—white flour

- 4 eggs

- 3 egg yolks

- 1 tablespoon lemon juice

- ½ teaspoon of cayenne pepper

- ½ teaspoon of paprika

- 1 tablespoon apple cider vinegar

- 2 tablespoons of unsalted butter.

Directions:

Slice the two toasted bread pieces in two, so you can end up with four pieces where each piece represents one serving. Take a large skillet or a pot and pour one cup of water in it. Add a tablespoon of vinegar and bring the water to boil. When the water starts to boil, break four eggs, one at a time, and poach the eggs by covering the skillet. Eggs should be done between 3 and 5 minutes of poaching, depending on how you like your eggs cooked. Next, place poached eggs on top of bread pieces. Take a skillet and add the butter so you could melt it, then add cayenne and paprika to the melted butter. Beat the egg yolks over medium heat, then add the eggs to the mixture with butter. Add lemon juice and whisk it into the egg and butter mixture. Once the sauce reaches an adequate thickness, remove from the heat, and pour over the eggs and toasted bread.

Nutrition:

- Potassium: 146mg

- Sodium: 206mg

- Phosphorus: 114mg

- Calories: 316.

6. Sweet Broiled Grapefruit

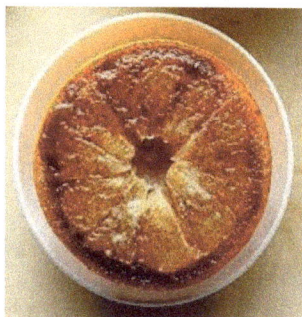

Preparation time: 5 minutes

Cooking time: 10 minutes

Serving: 2

Ingredients:

- 1 large grapefruit

- 2 tablespoons butter, softened

- 2 tablespoons sugar

- 1/2 teaspoon ground cinnamon.

Directions:

Preheat broiler. Cut around each grapefruit section to loosen fruit. Top with butter. Mix sugar and cinnamon; sprinkle over fruit.Place on a baking sheet. Broil 4 inches from heat until sugar is bubbly.

Nutrition: Calories: 203 Fat: 12g Saturated fat: 7g Cholesterol: 31mg Sodium: 116mg Carbohydrate: 26g Sugars: 24g Fiber: 2g 0 Protein: 1g.

7. French Toast with Applesauce

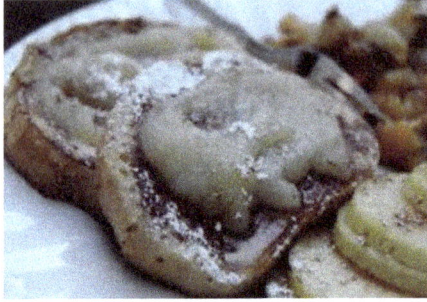

Preparation time: 10 minutes

Cooking time: 15 minutes

Servings: 4

Ingredients:

- ¼ cup unsweetened applesauce

- ½ cup milk

- 1 tsp. ground cinnamon

- 2 eggs

- 2 tbsp. white sugar

- 6 slices whole-wheat bread.

Directions:

Mix well applesauce, sugar, cinnamon, milk, and eggs in a mixing bowl. One slice at a time, soak the bread into the applesauce mixture until wet. On medium fire, heat a nonstick skillet greased with cooking spray. Add soaked bread one at a time and cook for 2-3 minutes per side or until lightly browned.

Serve and enjoy.

Nutrition:

- Calories per serving: 57

- Carbs: 6g

- Protein: 4g

- Fats: 4g

- Phosphorus: 69mg

- Potassium: 88mg

- Sodium: 43mg.

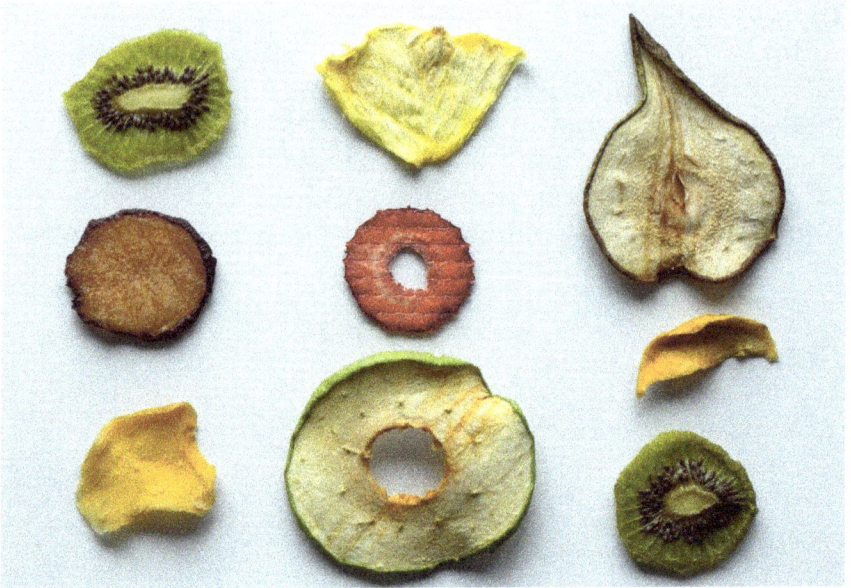

CHAPTER 6:

Meat Recipes

8. Pineapple and Mint Lamb Chops

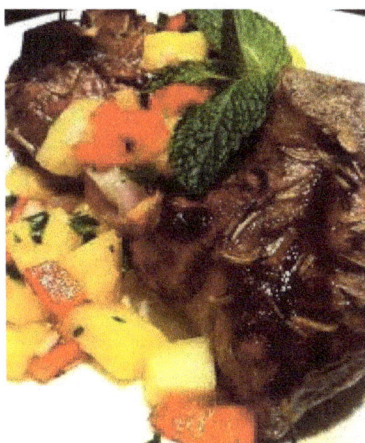

Preparation time: 10 minutes

Cooking time: 10 minutes

Servings: 4

Ingredients:

- 1/2 tablespoon olive oil
- 2 tablespoons pineapple juice
- ¼ tablespoon chopped fresh mint
- Salt and pepper to taste
- 4 lamb chops.

Directions:

Stir together olive oil, pineapple juice, and mint in a small bowl. Season with salt and pepper to taste. Place lamb chops in a shallow dish, and brush with the olive oil mixture. Marinate in the refrigerator for 1 hour.

Nutrition:

- Calories: 137

- Total Fat: 6.4g

- Cholesterol: 57mg

- Sodium: 49mg

- Total Carbohydrate: 0.8g

- Total Sugar: 0.7g

- Protein: 18g

- Calcium: 9mg

- Iron: 2mg

- Potassium: 230mg

- Phosphorus: 100mg.

9. Spiced Lamb Burgers

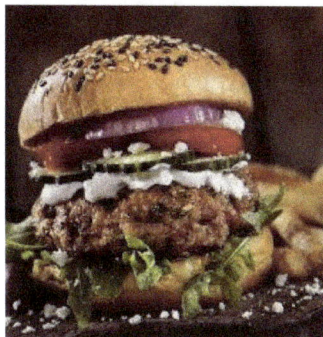

Preparation time: 10 minutes

Cooking time: 20 minutes

Servings: 2

Ingredients:

- 1 tbsp. extra virgin olive oil

- 1 tsp. cumin

- ½ finely diced red onion

- 1 minced garlic clove

- 1 tsp. harass spices

- 1 cup arugula

- 1 juiced lemon

- 6 oz. lean ground lamb

- 1 tbsp. parsley

- ½ cup low-fat plain yogurt.

Directions:

Preheat the broiler on a medium to high heat. Mix the ground lamb, red onion, parsley, harass spices, and olive oil until combined. Shape 1-inch thick patties using wet hands.

Add the patties to a baking tray and place under the broiler for 7-8 minutes on each side or until thoroughly cooked through. Mix the yogurt, lemon juice, and cumin and serve over the lamb burgers with a side salad of arugula.

Nutrition:

- Calories: 306 Fat: 20g

- Carbs: 10g Phosphorus: 269mg

- Potassium: 492mg Sodium: 86mg

- Protein: 23g.

10.   Roast Beef

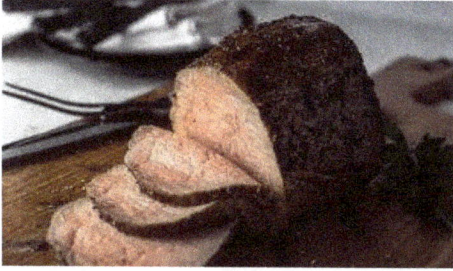

Preparation time: 25 minutes,

Cooking time: 55 minutes Serves: 3

Ingredients:

- Quality rump or sirloin tip roast.

Direction

Place in roasting pan on a shallow rack

Season with pepper and herbs

Insert meat thermometer in the center or thickest part of the roast

Roast to the desired degree of doneness

After removing from over for about 15 minutes, let it chill

In the end, the roast should be moist.

Nutrition: Calories: 158 Protein: 24g Fat: 6g Carbs: 0gPhosphorus: 206mg Potassium: 328mg Sodium: 55mg.

11.   Pork Peccadillo

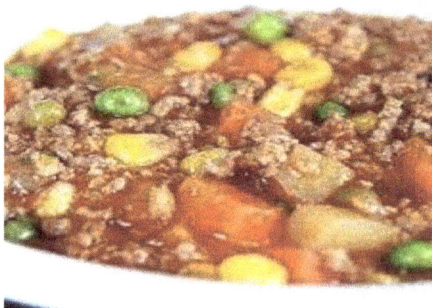

Preparation time: 15 minutes

Cooking time: 20 minutes

Servings: 4

Ingredients:

- 2 tablespoons olive oil
- 1 onion, diced, 2 cloves garlic, crushed
- 2 1/2 pounds ground pork
- Salt and pepper to taste
- 1 yellow bell pepper, cut into thin strips
- 1 green bell pepper, cut into thin strips
- 1 red bell pepper, cut into thin strips
- ½ cup kale, chopped.

Directions:

Heat the olive oil in a large skillet over medium heat. Cook and stir the onion and garlic in the oil until tender, about 5 minutes. Remove the onion and garlic from the pan and set aside.

Crumble the pork into the skillet and cook until no longer pink. Return the onion and garlic to the skillet and stir through the pork. Season with salt and pepper. Cover the skillet and cook the mixture for 5 minutes.

Stir the green bell pepper, red bell pepper, yellow bell pepper into the mixture; cover and cook another 5 minutes. Add the kale to the skillet and stir just before serving.

Nutrition:

- Calories: 163 Total Fat: 9g

- Saturated Fat: 1.6g

- Cholesterol: 39mg Sodium: 36mg

- Total Carbohydrate: 6.2g

- Protein: 14.9g Calcium: 26mg

- Iron: 1mg

- Potassium: 367mg

- Phosphorus: 241mg.

12.   Steak and Broccoli Salad

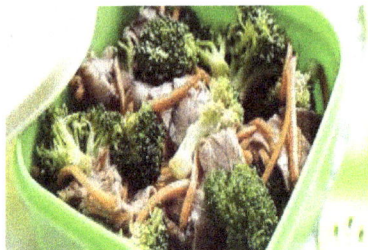

Preparation time: 5 minutes

Cooking time: 10 minutes

Servings: 4

Ingredients:

- ½ cup fresh kale, rinsed and dried
- 1/2 cup dried cranberries
- 1-1/2 cup chopped broccoli
- ½ pound top round steak, thinly sliced
- 1 pinch ground black pepper.

Directions:

Arrange kale on a large plate. Sprinkle with cranberries. Set aside. In a non-stick skillet, cook steak over medium heat until no pink remains, and steak is thoroughly cooked, then add broccoli.

Arrange cooked steak over salad. Sprinkle salt and pepper on top.

Nutrition: Calories: 199 Total Fat: 11.1gSaturated Fat: 1.2g, Cholesterol: 18mgSodium: 96mgTotal Carbohydrate: 13.3gProtein: 13.5gCalcium: 148mgIron: 3mgPotassium: 693mg Phosphorus: 300mg.

13.   Country Fried Steak

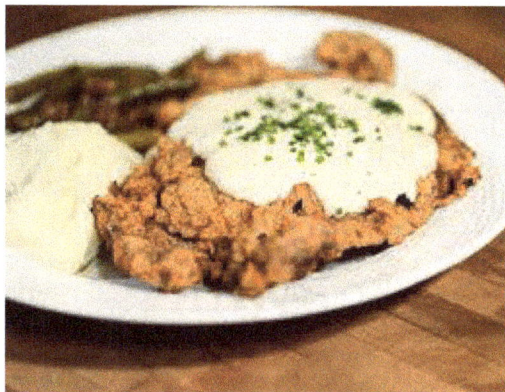

Preparation time: 10 minutes

Cook time: 100 minutes

Servings: 3

Ingredients:

- 1 large onion

- ½ cup flour

- 3 tbsps. Vegetable oil

- ¼ tsp. pepper

- 1½ lbs. round steak

- ½ tsp. paprika.

Directions:

Trim excess fat from steak.

Cut into small pieces.

Combine flour, paprika, and pepper and mix together.

Preheat skillet with oil.

Cook steak on both sides.

When the color of steak is brown, remove to a platter.

Add water (150 ml) and stir around the skillet.

Return browned steak to skillet, if necessary, add water again so that bottom side of steak does not stick.

Nutrition:

- Calories: 248

- Protein: 30g

- Fat: 10g

- Carbs: 5g

- Phosphorus: 190mg

- Potassium: 338mg

- Sodium: 60mg.

14.   Sweet and Spicy Braised Beef

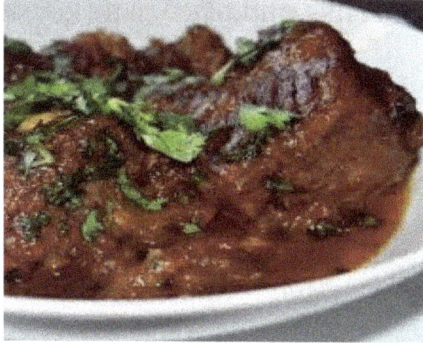

Preparation time: 20 minutes

Cooking time: 7 hours 5 minutes

Servings: 4

Ingredients:

- 1-pound beef, well-trimmed
- 4 ounces apple juice
- 1 medium onion, thinly sliced into half moons
- 1 tablespoon honey
- 1 tablespoon chili powder
- 1 teaspoon cumin
- 1 teaspoon dried thyme
- 1 teaspoon black pepper
- 1 tablespoon olive oil
- 2 tablespoon cornstarch.

Directions:

Place sliced onion in a slow cooker.

In large deep skillet, heat oil and brown beef on all sides.

Remove beef from skillet and place in a slow cooker.

Add apple juice and spices to the pan. Loosen browned bits from the bottom of the pan with a spatula.

Allow the juice to simmer until reduced by approximately half.

Pour juice over beef in the slow cooker. Set slow cooker on low and cook for approximately 7 hours.

Remove beef from slow cooker to a deep platter or serving bowl. Shred using two forks.

Pour the juice into a medium saucepan. Bring to simmer.

Pour sauce over meat and serve.

Nutrition:

- Calories: 302

- Saturated Fat: 2.3g

- Cholesterol: 75mg

- Sodium: 82mg

- Total Carbohydrate: 32.4g

- Protein: 25.5g

- Calcium: 48mg

- Potassium: 283mg

- Phosphorus: 125mg.

CHAPTER 7:

Seafood Mains

15.   Shrimp Paella

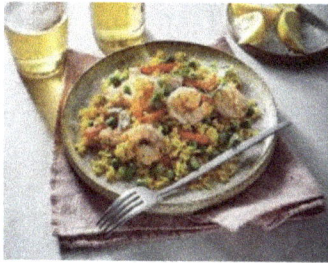

Preparation time: 5 minutes

Cooking time: 10 minutes

Servings: 2

Ingredients:

- 1 cup cooked brown rice

- 1 chopped red onion

- 1 tsp. paprika

- 1 chopped garlic clove

- 1 tbsp. olive oil

- 6 oz. frozen cooked shrimp

- 1 deseeded and sliced chili pepper

- 1 tbsp. oregano.

Directions:

Heat the olive oil in a large pan on medium-high heat.

Add the onion and garlic and sauté for 2-3 minutes until soft.

Now add the shrimp and sauté for a further 5 minutes or until hot through.

Now add the herbs, spices, chili, and rice with 1/2 cup boiling water.

Stir until everything is warm, and the water has been absorbed.

Plate up and serve.

Nutrition:

- Calories: 221

- Protein: 17g

- Sodium: 235mg

- Potassium: 176mg

- Phosphorus: 189mg.

16. Salmon & Pesto Salad

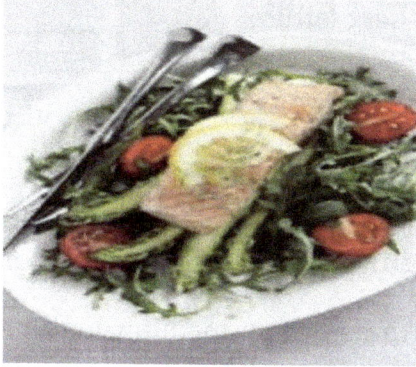

Preparation time: 5 minutes

Cooking time: 15 minutes

Servings: 2

Ingredients:

- For the pesto: 1 minced garlic clove
- ½ cup fresh arugula
- ¼ cup extra virgin olive oil l
- ½ cup fresh basil
- 1 tsp. black pepper
- For the salmon:
- 4 oz. skinless salmon fillet
- 1 tbsp. coconut oil.

For the salad:

- ½ juiced lemon

- 2 sliced radishes

- ½ cup iceberg lettuce

- 1 tsp. black pepper.

Directions:

Prepare the pesto by blending all the pesto ingredients in a food processor or by grinding with a pestle and mortar. Set aside.

Add a skillet to the stove on medium-high heat and melt the coconut oil.

Add the salmon to the pan.

Cook for 7-8 minutes and turn over.

Cook for a further 3-4 minutes or until cooked through.

Remove fillets from the skillet and allow to rest.

Mix the lettuce and the radishes and squeeze over the juice of ½ lemon.

Flake the salmon with a fork and mix through the salad.

Toss to coat and sprinkle with a little black pepper to serve.

Nutrition:

- Calories: 221 Protein: 13g

- Carbs: 1g Fat: 34g

- Sodium: 80mg

- Potassium: 119mg

- Phosphorus: 158mg.

17.   **Baked Fennel & Garlic Sea Bass**

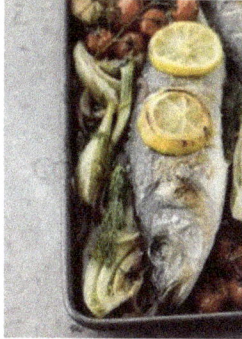

Preparation time: 5 minutes

Cooking time: 15 minutes

Servings: 2

Ingredients:

- 1 lemon

- ½ sliced fennel bulb

- 6 oz. sea bass fillets

- 1 tsp. black pepper

- 2 garlic cloves.

Directions:

Preheat the oven to 375°F/Gas mark 5. Sprinkle black pepper over the Sea Bass. Slice the fennel bulb and garlic cloves. Add 1 salmon fillet and half the fennel and garlic to one sheet of baking paper or tin foil. Squeeze in 1/2 lemon juices. Repeat for the other fillet. Fold and add to the oven for 12-15 minutes or until fish is thoroughly cooked through.

Meanwhile, add boiling water to your couscous, cover, and allow to steam.

Serve with your choice of rice or salad.

Nutrition:

- Calories: 221

- Protein: 14g

- Carbs: 3g

- Fat: 2g

- Sodium: 119mg

- Potassium: 398mg

- Phosphorus: 149mg.

18. Oregano Salmon With Crunchy Crust

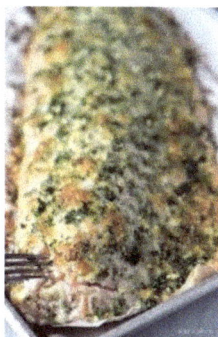

Preparation time: 10 minutes

Cooking time: 2 hoursServings: 2

Ingredients:

- 8 oz. salmon fillet

- 2 tablespoons panko breadcrumbs

- 1 oz. Parmesan, grated

- 1 teaspoon dried oregano

- 1 teaspoon sunflower oil.

Directions:

In the mixing bowl, combine together panko breadcrumbs, Parmesan, and dried oregano. Sprinkle the salmon with olive oil and coat in the breadcrumb's mixture. After this, line the baking tray with baking paper. Place the salmon in the tray and transfer in the preheated to the 385F oven. Bake the salmon for 25 minutes.

Nutrition: Calories: 245 Fat: 12.8g Fiber: 0.6g Carbs: 5.9g Protein: 27.5g.

19.   Sardine Fish Cakes

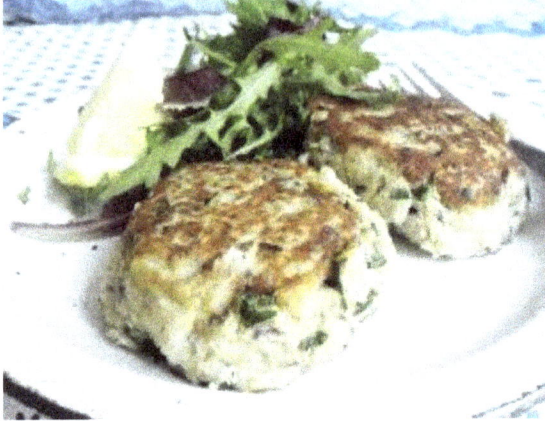

Preparation time: 10 minutes

Cooking time: 10 minutes

Servings: 4

Ingredients:

- 11 oz. sardines, canned, drained

- 1/3 cup shallot, chopped

- 1 teaspoon chili flakes

- ½ teaspoon salt

- 2 tablespoon wheat flour, whole grain

- 1 egg, beaten

- 1 tablespoon chives, chopped

- 1 teaspoon olive oil

- 1 teaspoon butter.

Directions:

Put the butter in the skillet and melt it.

Add shallot and cook it until translucent.

After this, transfer the shallot to the mixing bowl.

Add sardines, chili flakes, salt, flour, egg, chives, and mix up until smooth with the help of the fork. Make the medium size cakes and place them in the skillet. Add olive oil. Roast the fish cakes for 3 minutes from each side over the medium heat.

Dry the cooked fish cakes with the paper towel if needed and transfer to the serving plates.

Nutrition:

- Calories: 221

- Fat: 12.2g

- Fiber: 0.1g

- Carbs: 5.4g

- Protein: 21.3g.

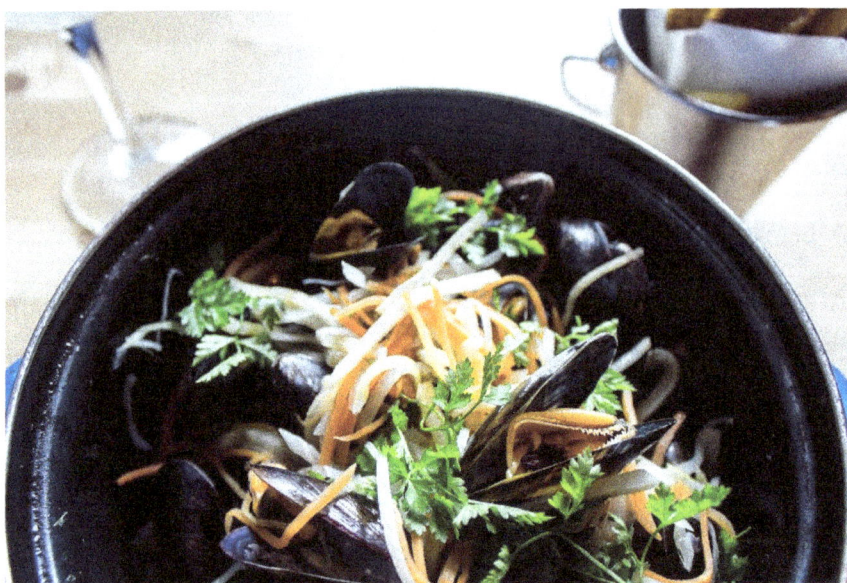

CHAPTER 8:

Vegetarian Recipes

20.   Tofu Stir Fry

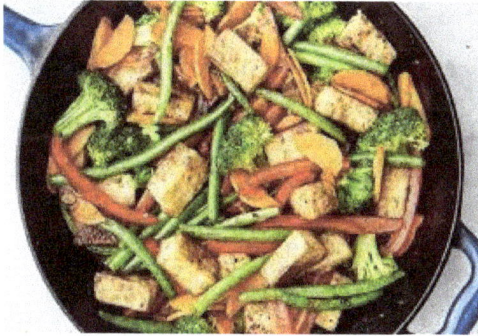

Preparation time: 15 minutes

Cooking time: 20 minutes

Servings: 4
Ingredients:

- 1 teaspoon sugar

- 1 tablespoon lime juice

- 1 tablespoon low sodium soy sauce

- 2 tablespoons cornstarch

- 2 egg whites, beaten

- 1/2 cup unseasoned bread crumbs

- 1 tablespoon vegetable oil

- 16 ounces tofu, cubed

- 1 clove garlic, minced

- 1 tablespoon sesame oil

- 1 red bell pepper, sliced into strips

- 1 cup broccoli florets

- 1 teaspoon herb seasoning blend

- Dash black pepper

- Sesame seeds

- Steamed white rice.

Directions:

Dissolve sugar in a mixture of lime juice and soy sauce. Set aside. In the first bowl, put the cornstarch. Add the egg whites to the second bowl. Place the breadcrumbs in the third bowl. Dip each tofu cubes in the first, second, and third bowls. Pour vegetable oil into a pan over medium heat. Cook tofu cubes until golden. Drain the tofu and set aside. Remove the oil from the pan and add sesame oil. Add garlic, bell pepper, and broccoli. Cook until crisp-tender. Season with the seasoning blend and pepper. Put the tofu back and toss to mix. Pour soy sauce mixture on top and transfer to serving bowls. Garnish with the sesame seeds and serve on top of white rice.

Nutrition: Calories: 401 Protein: 19gSodium: 584mg Potassium: 317mg Phosphorus: 177mg Calcium: 253mg.

21. **Broccoli Pancake**

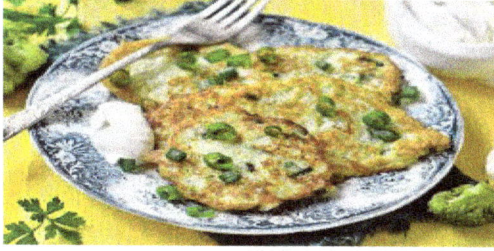

Preparation time: 10 minutes

Cooking time: 5 minutes

Servings: 4
Ingredients:

- 3 cups broccoli florets, diced

- 2 eggs, beaten

- 2 tablespoons all-purpose flour

- 1/2 cup onion, chopped

- 2 tablespoons olive oil.

Directions:

Boil broccoli in water for 5 minutes. Drain and set aside. Mix egg and flour. Add onion and broccoli to the mixture.

Cook the broccoli pancake until brown on both sides.

Nutrition:

- Calories: 140 Protein: 6 g

- Sodium: 58mgPotassium: 276mg

- Phosphorus: 101mg.

22.   **Carrot Casserole**

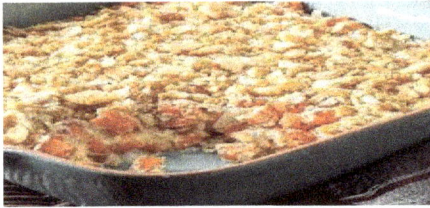

Preparation time: 10 minutes

Cooking time: 20 minutes Serving: 8
Ingredients:

- 1-pound carrots, sliced into rounds

- 12 low-sodium crackers

- 2 tablespoons butter

- 2 tablespoons onion, chopped

- 1/4 cup cheddar cheese, shredded.

Directions:

Preheat your oven to 350 degrees F.

Boil carrots in a pot of water until tender.

Drain the carrots and reserve ¼ cup liquid.

Mash carrots. Add all the ingredients into the carrots except cheese. Place the mashed carrots in a casserole dish.

Sprinkle cheese on top and bake in the oven for 15 minutes.

Nutrition: Calories: 97 Protein: 2gSodium: 174mg Potassium: 153mg.

23. **Eggplant Fries**

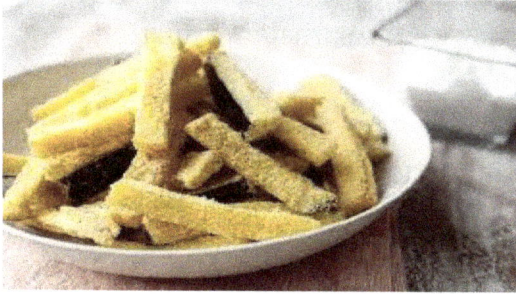

Preparation time: 10 minutes

Cooking time: 5 minutes

Servings: 6
Ingredients:

- 2 eggs, beaten

- 1 cup almond milk

- 1 teaspoon hot sauce

- 3/4 cup cornstarch

- 3 teaspoons dry ranch seasoning mix

- 3/4 cup dry bread crumbs

- 1 eggplant, sliced into strips

- 1/2 cup oil.

Directions:

In a bowl, mix eggs, milk, and hot sauce.

In a dish, mix cornstarch, seasoning, and breadcrumbs.

Dip first the eggplant strips in the egg mixture.

Coat each strip with the cornstarch mixture.

Pour oil into a pan over medium heat.

Once hot, add the fries and cook for 3 minutes or until golden.

Nutrition:

- Calories: 234

- Protein: 7g

- Sodium: 212mg

- Potassium: 215mg

- Phosphorus: 86mg

- Calcium: 70mg.

24.   Grilled Squash

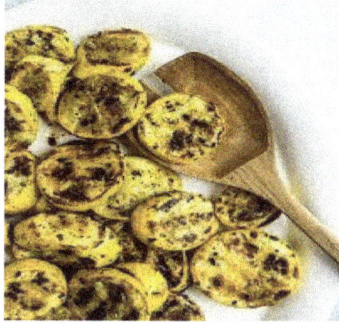

Preparation time: 10 minutes

Cooking time: 6 minutes

Servings: 8

Ingredients:

- 4 zucchinis, rinsed, drained, and sliced

- 4 crookneck squash, rinsed, drained, and sliced

- Cooking spray

- 1/4 teaspoon garlic powder

- 1/4 teaspoon black pepper.

Directions:

Arrange squash on a baking sheet. Spray with oil. Season with garlic powder and pepper. Grill for 3 minutes per side or until tender but not too soft.

Nutrition: Calories: 17Protein: 1gPotassium: 262mg Phosphorus: 39mg Calcium: 16mgFiber: 1.1 g.

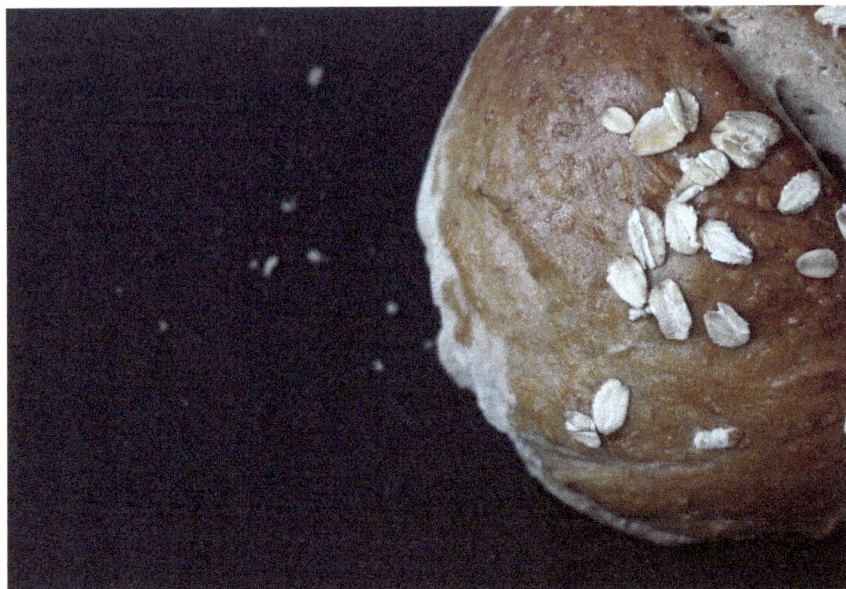

CHAPTER 9:

Salads Recipes

25.   Balsamic Beet Salad

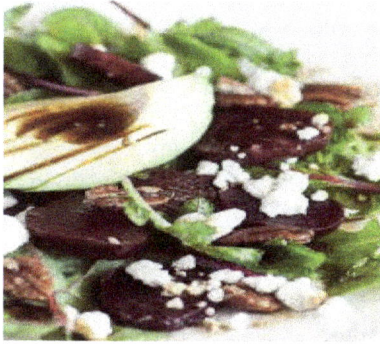

Preparation time: 10 minutes

Cooking time: 0 minutes

Servings: 2

Ingredients:

- 1 cucumber, peeled and sliced

- 15 oz. canned low-sodium beets, sliced

- 4 teaspoon balsamic vinegar

- 2 teaspoon sesame oil

- 2 tablespoons Gorgonzola cheese.

Directions:

Take a suitable salad bowl.

Start tossing in all the ingredients.

Mix well and serve.

Nutrition:

- Calories: 145

- Sodium: 426mg

- Carbohydrate: 16.4g

- Protein: 5g

- Phosphorous: 79mg

- Potassium: 229mg.

26.   Shrimp Salad

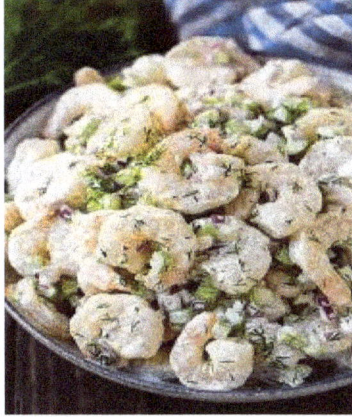

Preparation time: 10 minutes

Cooking time: 0 minutes

Servings: 4

Ingredients:

- 1 lb. shrimp, boiled and chopped

- 1 hardboiled egg, chopped

- 1 tablespoon celery, chopped

- 1 tablespoon green pepper, chopped

- 1 tablespoon onion, chopped

- 2 tablespoons mayonnaise

- 1 teaspoon lemon juice

- ½ teaspoon chili powder

- ⅛ Teaspoon hot sauce

- ½ teaspoon dry mustard

- Lettuce, chopped or shredded.

Directions:

Take a suitable salad bowl.

Start tossing in all the ingredients.

Mix well and serve.

Nutrition:

- Calories: 184

- Sodium: 381mg

- Carbohydrate: 4.3g

- Protein: 27.5g

- Phosphorous: 249mg

- Potassium: 233mg.

27. Chicken Cranberry Sauce Salad

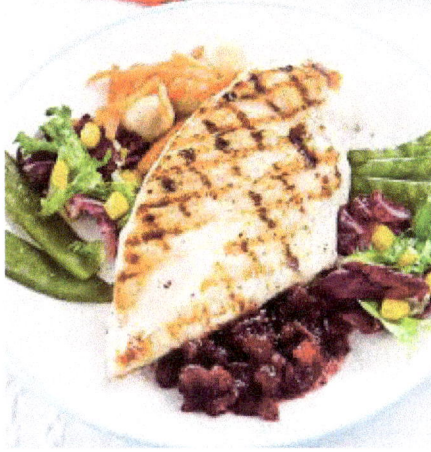

Preparation time: 10 minutes

Cooking time: 0 minutes

Servings: 6

Ingredients:

- 3 cups of chicken meat, cooked, cubed

- 1 cup grapes

- 2 cups carrots, shredded

- 1/4 red onion, chopped

- 1 large yellow bell pepper, chopped

- 1/4 cup mayonnaise

- 1/2 cup cranberry sauce.

Directions:

Put all the salad ingredients into a suitable salad bowl.

Toss them well and refrigerate for 1 hour.

Serve.

Nutrition:

- Calories: 240 Sodium: 161mg

- Carbohydrate: 19.4g

- Protein: 21g

- Calcium: 31mg

- Phosphorous: 260mg

- Potassium: 351mg.

28.   Egg Celery Salad

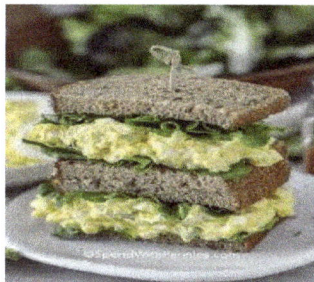

Preparation time: 10 minutes

Cooking time: 0 minutes Servings: 4

Ingredients:

- 4 eggs, boiled, peeled, and chopped

- 1/4 cup celery, chopped

- 1/2 cup sweet onion, chopped

- 2 tablespoons sweet pickle, chopped

- 3 tablespoons mayonnaise

- 1 tablespoon mustard.

Directions:

Put all the salad ingredients into a suitable salad bowl.

Toss them well and refrigerate for 1 hour. Serve.

Nutrition: Calories: 134Sodium: 259mg   Protein: 6.8g
Phosphorous: 357mg Potassium: 113mg.

29. Almond Pasta Salad

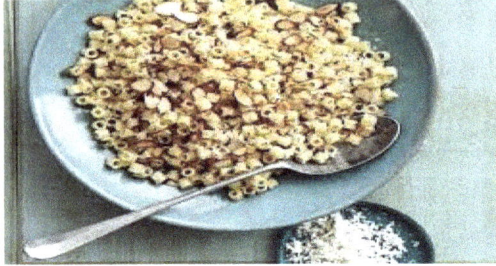

Preparation time: 10 minutes

Cooking time: 0 minutes

Servings: 14

Ingredients:

- 1 lb. elbow macaroni, cooked

- 1/2 cup sun-dried tomatoes, diced

- 1 (15 oz.) can whole artichokes, diced

- 1 orange bell pepper, diced

- 3 green onions, sliced

- 2 tablespoons basil, sliced

- 2 oz. slivered almonds.

Dressing:

- 1 garlic clove, minced

- 1 tablespoon Dijon mustard

- 1 tablespoon raw honey

- 1/4 cup white balsamic vinegar

- 1/3 cup olive oil.

Directions:

Take a suitable salad bowl.

Start tossing in all the ingredients.

Mix well and serve.

Nutrition:

- Calories: 260

- Sodium: 143mg

- Carbohydrate: 41.4g

- Protein: 9.6g

- Calcium: 44mg

- Phosphorous: 39mg

- Potassium: 585mg.

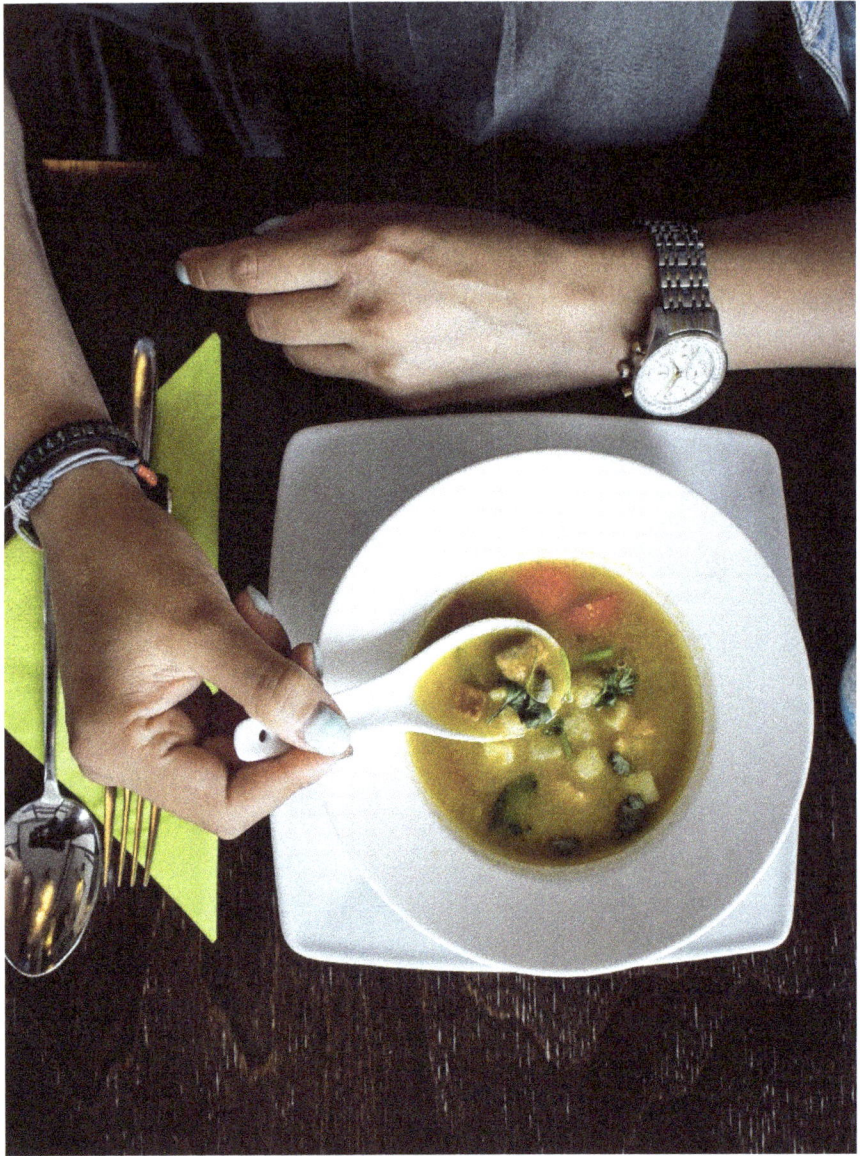

CHAPTER 10:

Soups and Stews

30.   Spaghetti Squash & Yellow Bell-Pepper Soup

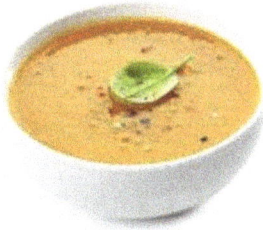

Preparation time: 10 minutes

Cooking time: 45 minutes

Servings: 4

Ingredients:

- 2 diced yellow bell peppers

- 2 chopped large garlic cloves

- 1 peeled and cubed spaghetti squash

- 1 quartered and sliced onion

- 1 tbsp. dried thyme

- 1 tbsp. coconut oil

- 1 tsp. curry powder

- 4 cups water.

Directions:

Heat the oil in a large pan over medium-high heat before sweating the onions and garlic for 3-4 minutes. Sprinkle over the curry powder. Add the stock and bring to a boil over a high heat before adding the squash, pepper, and thyme. Turn down the heat, cover, and allow to simmer for 25-30 minutes. Continue to simmer until squash is soft if needed. Allow to cool before blitzing in a blender/food processor until smooth.

Serve!

Nutrition:

- Calories: 103

- Protein: 2g

- Carbs: 17g

- Fat: 4g

- Sodium: (Na) 32mg

- Potassium: (K) 365mg

- Phosphorus: 50mg.

31.   **Red Pepper & Brie Soup**

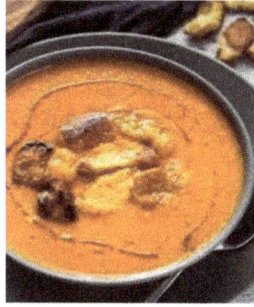

Preparation time: 10 minutes

Cooking time: 35 minutes

Servings: 4

Ingredients:

- 1 tsp. paprika

- 1 tsp. cumin

- 1 chopped red onion

- 2 chopped garlic cloves

- ¼ cup crumbled brie

- 2 tbsps. extra virgin olive oil

- 4 chopped red bell peppers

- 4 cups water.

Directions:

Heat the oil in a pot over medium heat. Sweat the onions and peppers for 5 minutes. Add the garlic cloves, cumin, and paprika and sauté for 3-4 minutes. Add the water and allow it to boil before turning the heat down to simmer for 30 minutes.

Remove from the heat and allow to cool slightly. Put the mixture in a food processor and blend until smooth. Pour into serving bowls and add the crumbled brie to the top with a little black pepper.

Enjoy!

Nutrition:

- Calories: 152 Protein: 3g

- Carbs: 8g Fat: 11g

- Sodium: 66mg

- Potassium: 270mg

- Phosphorus: 207mg.

32. **Turkey & Lemongrass Soup**

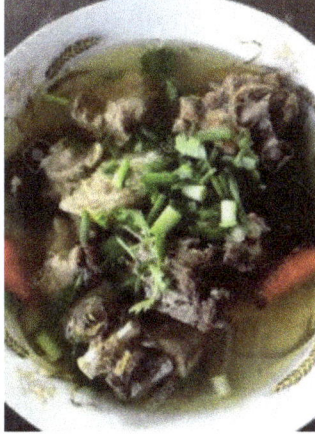

Preparation time: 5 minutes

Cooking time: 40 minutes

Servings: 4
Ingredients:

- 1 fresh lime

- ¼ cup fresh basil leaves

- 1 tbsp. cilantro

- 1 cup canned and drained water chestnuts

- 1 tbsp. coconut oil

- 1 thumb-size minced ginger piece

- 2 chopped scallions

- 1 finely chopped green chili

- 4oz. skinless and sliced turkey breasts

- 1 minced garlic clove, minced

- ½ finely sliced stick lemongrass

- 1 chopped white onion, chopped

- 4 cups water.

Directions:

Crush the lemongrass, cilantro, chili, 1 tbsp. oil and basil leaves in a blender or pestle and mortar to form a paste.

Heat a large pan/wok with 1 tbsp. olive oil on high heat.

Sauté the onions, garlic, and ginger until soft.

Add the turkey and brown each side for 4-5 minutes.

Add the broth and stir.

Now add the paste and stir.

Next, add the water chestnuts, turn down the heat slightly and allow to simmer for 25-30 minutes or until turkey is thoroughly cooked through.

Serve hot with the green onion sprinkled over the top.

Nutrition:

- Calories: 123 Protein: 10g

- Carbs: 12g Fat: 3g

- Sodium: 501mg

- Potassium: 151mg

- Phosphorus: 110mg.

33. **Paprika Pork Soup**

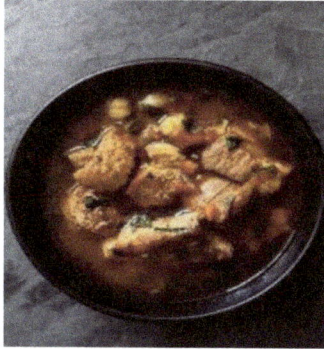

Preparation time: 10 minutes

Cooking time: 35 minutes

Servings: 4

Ingredients:

- 4 oz. sliced pork loin

- 1 tsp. black pepper

- 2 minced garlic cloves

- 1 cup baby spinach

- 3 cups water

- 1 tbsp. extra-virgin olive oil

- 1 chopped onion

- 1 tbsp. paprika.

Directions:

In a large pot, add the oil, chopped onion, and minced garlic.

Sauté for 5 minutes on low heat.

Add the pork slices to the onions and cook for 7-8 minutes or until browned.

Add the water to the pan and bring to a boil on high heat.

Season with pepper to serve.

Nutrition:

- Calories: 165

- Protein: 13g

- Carbs: 10g

- Fat: 9g

- Sodium: 269mg

- Potassium: 486mg

- Phosphorus: 158mg.

34.   Mediterranean Vegetable Soup

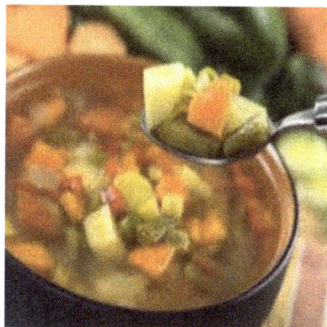

Preparation time: 5 minutes

Cooking time: 30 minutes

Servings: 4

Ingredients:

1 tbsp. oregano

2 minced garlic cloves

1 tsp. black pepper

1 diced zucchini

1 cup diced eggplant

4 cups water

1 diced red pepper

1 tbsp. extra-virgin olive oil

1 diced red onion.

Directions:

Soak the vegetables in warm water prior to use.

In a large pot, add the oil, chopped onion, and minced garlic.

Sweat for 5 minutes on low heat.

Add the other vegetables to the onions and cook for 7-8 minutes.

Add the stock to the pan and bring to a boil on high heat.

Stir in the herbs, reduce the heat, and simmer for a further 20 minutes or until thoroughly cooked through.

Season with pepper to serve.

Nutrition:

- Calories: 152

- Protein: 1g

- Carbs: 6g

- Fat: 3g

- Sodium: 3mg

- Potassium: 229mg

- Phosphorus: 45mg.

CHAPTER 11:

Snacks Recipes

35.   Pineapple Cabbage Coleslaw

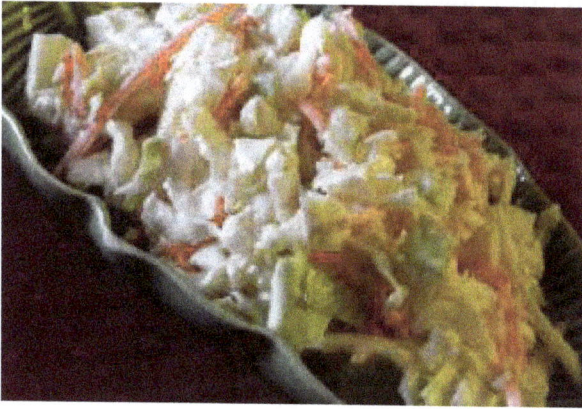

Preparation time: 10 minutes

Cooking time: 0 minutes

Servings: 12

Ingredients:

- 12 oz. (bag) broccoli coleslaw

- 12 oz. Napa cabbage, finely shredded

- 20 oz. (can) unsweetened pineapple, drained

- 1/2 cup green onions, sliced

- 1 cup mayonnaise

- 1 tablespoon seasoned rice vinegar

- 1 teaspoon coarse ground black pepper.

Directions:

Toss the cabbage with the broccoli and all the other ingredients in a salad bowl.

Refrigerate this coleslaw for at least 1 hour.

Serve.

Nutrition:

- Calories: 186

- Total Fat: 12.7g

- Saturated Fat: 2g

- Cholesterol: 5mg

- Sodium: 224mg

- Carbohydrate: 18g

- Protein: 2g

- Calcium: 42mg

- Phosphorous: 106mg

- Potassium: 139mg.

36.   **Seafood Croquettes**

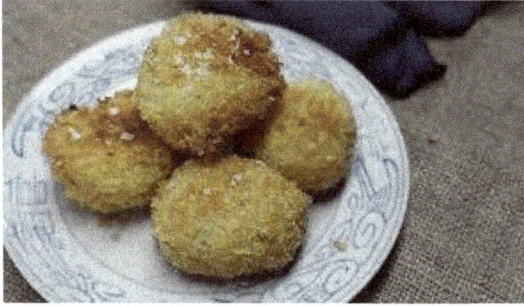

Preparation time: 10 minutes

Cooking time: 20 minutes

Servings: 8

Ingredients:

- 14.75 oz. packed salmon

- 2 egg whites

- ¼ cup chopped onion

- ½ teaspoon black pepper

- ½ cup plain breadcrumbs

- 2 tablespoons lemon juice

- ½ teaspoon ground mustard

- ¼ cup regular mayonnaise.

Directions:

Drain the packed salmon and transfer it to a bowl. Stir in all the other ingredients except the oil and mix well. Make 8 patties out of this mixture and keep them aside. Add the oil to a pan and place it over medium-high heat. Add 4 patties at a time and sear them for 3 minutes per side. Cook the remaining four in the same manner until golden brown. Serve.

Nutrition:

- Calories: 282 Total Fat: 12g

- Saturated Fat: 2.6g

- Cholesterol: 66mg

- Sodium: 202mg Carbohydrate: 7.4g

- Protein: 12.6g Calcium: 88mg

- Phosphorous: 137mg

- Potassium: 253mg.

37.   Herbed Shrimp Spread

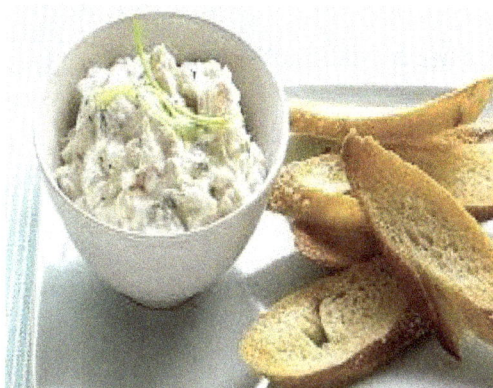

Preparation time: 10 minutes

Cooking time: 0 minutes

Servings: 8

Ingredients:

- 1/2 lb. shrimp, cooked, peeled, and deveined

- 1/2 cup reduced-fat sour cream

- 1/2 cup light mayonnaise

- 2 scallions, coarsely chopped

- 1 teaspoon lemon zest, finely grated

- 2 teaspoons fresh lemon juice

- 1/4 cup parsley, chopped.

Directions:

Begin by tossing the minced shrimp with the sour cream in a bowl.

Add in the mayonnaise, scallions, and lemon juice, and lemon zest.

Mix well and garnish with parsley.

Serve the spread.

Nutrition:

- Calories: 118

- Total Fat: 8.3g

- Saturated Fat: 2.7g

- Cholesterol: 65mg

- Sodium: 177mg

- Carbohydrate: 4.6g

- Protein: 6.7g

- Calcium: 35mg

- Phosphorous: 203mg

- Potassium: 95mg.

38.   Almond Caramel Corn

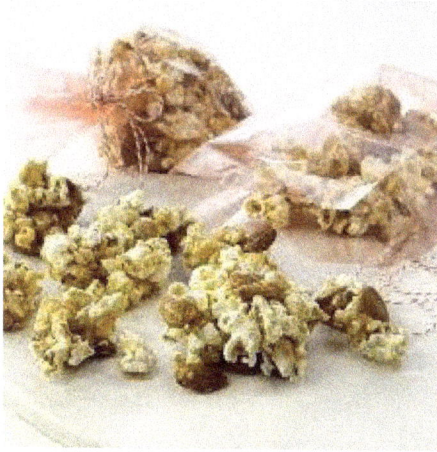

Preparation time: 10 minutes

Cooking time: 1 hour 15 minutes

Servings: 30

Ingredients:

- 12 cups popped popcorn

- 3 cups unbranched whole almonds

- 1 cup brown Swerve

- ½ cup butter

- ¼ cup light corn syrup

- ½ teaspoon baking soda.

Directions:

Take a suitable roasting pan and spread the almonds and popcorn in it.

Whisk the Swerve with the butter and corn syrup in a heavy saucepan.

Stir-fry this corn syrup for about 5 minutes up to a boil, then add in the baking soda.

Pour this corn sauce over the popcorn and almonds in the pan.

Bake the popcorn mixture for approximately 1 hour at 200 degrees F in the oven.

Stir well, then serve.

Nutrition:

- Calories: 120 Total Fat: 8g

- Saturated Fat: 2.3g

- Cholesterol: 8mg

- Sodium: 45mg

- Carbohydrate: 6.5g

- Calcium: 31mg

- Phosphorous: 23mg

- Potassium: 88mg.

39.   Sweet Popped Popcorn

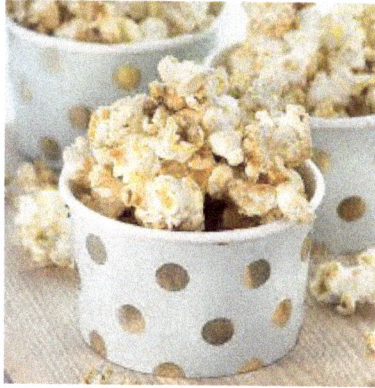

Preparation time: 10 minutes

Cooking time: 5 minutes

Servings: 4

Ingredients:

- 2 ¾ oz. popped popcorn
- 2 tablespoons butter
- 2 tablespoons corn syrup
- 2 tablespoons brown Swerve
- 1 teaspoon oil.

Directions:

Whisk the corn syrup, brown Swerve, and oil in a saucepan.

Stir-fry the corn syrup mixture for 5 minutes, then remove it from heat.

Add the butter and mix well, then let the mixture cool.

Toss in the popped popcorn.

Serve.

Nutrition:

- Calories: 224

- Total Fat: 7.1g

- Sodium: 178mg

- Protein: 1.2g

- Calcium: 8g

- Phosphorous: 11mg

- Potassium: 38mg.

40.   Spiced Tortilla Chips

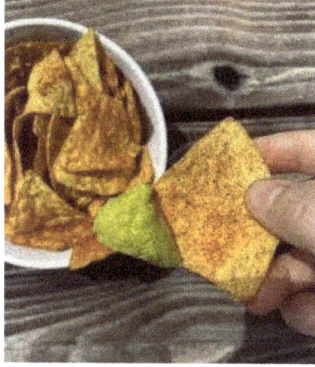

Preparation time: 10 minutes

Cooking time: 8 minutes

Servings: 8

Ingredients:

- 4 (12-inch) flour tortillas, cut into wedges

- 4 tablespoons olive oil

- ½ teaspoon paprika

- ½ teaspoon rosemary seasoning

- ½ teaspoon cayenne pepper

- Parmesan cheese.

Directions:

Begin by switching the oven to 425 degrees F to preheat. Grease the baking sheet with cooking spray. Add all the spices and cheese to a small bowl. Mix well and keep this mixture aside. Cut the tortillas into 8 wedges and coat them with the cheese mixture. Spread them on a baking tray and drizzle the remaining cheese mixture on top. Bake for about 8 minutes at 350 degrees F in a preheated oven. Serve fresh.

Nutrition:

- Calories: 87

- Sodium: 5mg

- Carbohydrate: 5.5g

- Dietary Fiber: 0.8g

- Sugars 0.1g

- Protein: 0.7g

- Calcium: 10mg

- Phosphorous: 79mg

- Potassium: 28mg.

41.   Date and Blueberry Muffins

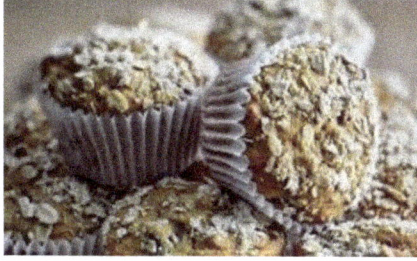

Preparation time: 20 minutes

Cooking time: 15 minutes

Servings: 12

Ingredients:

- 2 tablespoons flax meal

- 6 tablespoons water

- 1 cup almond flour

- 1 cup coconut flour

- 2 teaspoons baking soda

- 1 teaspoon sea salt

- 2 tablespoons mixed spice

- 1 cup dates, pitted

- 2 cups canned pumpkin

- 1 teaspoon lemon juice

- ¼ cup coconut oil

- 5 ounces frozen blueberries

- ¾ cup zucchini, grated

- ¾ cup chopped walnuts.

Directions:

Preheat oven to 350° F.

Line 12 muffin cups with paper liners.

Mix together the flax meal and water and leave for a few minutes until it becomes a gel-like consistency.

Mix almond flour, coconut flour, baking soda, sea salt, and mixed spice in a large bowl. Set aside.

In a food processor, pulse together the pitted dates, pumpkin, and lemon juice together with the flax water and coconut oil.

Mix the pumpkin mixture into the dry ingredients. Mix well.

Gently stir in the blueberries, grated zucchini, and walnuts.

Divide the mixture evenly between the prepared muffin cups.

Bake for about 30 minutes. If the muffins are too gooey, after this time, leave for a few minutes longer.

Nutrition:

- Calories: 211

- Fat: 12.0g

- Carbs: 23.3g

- Dietary Fiber: 7.2g

- Protein: 5.0g.

42. Cranberry and Lemon Cookies

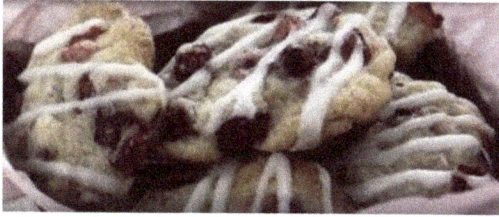

Preparation time: 10 minutes

Cooking time: 20 minutes

Servings: 12

Ingredients:

- ½ cup coconut milk

- 1 tablespoon ground flaxseed

- 1¼ cups brown organic superfine sugar

- ½ cup unsweetened apple sauce

- ¼ cup vegetable oil

- 1 tablespoon fresh lemon juice

- 1½ teaspoons lemon zest

- 2 teaspoons vanilla extract

- 1¼ cups unbleached general-purpose flour

- 1 cup whole wheat flour

- 1 teaspoon baking soda

- ½ teaspoon salt

- 1 cup dried cranberries

- 1 cup chopped walnuts.

Directions:

Preheat the oven to 350°F.

Prepare 2 cookie sheets with parchment paper.

Warm the coconut milk and stir in the flaxseed. Leave to one side for it to gel.

In a large bowl, stir together all of the wet ingredients with the sugar. Stir in the gelled flax seed.

In another bowl, sift together the flours, baking soda, and salt.

Add the flour mix to the wet ingredients a little at a time until fully combined.

When a dough has formed, stir in the nuts and cranberries.

Using a spoon, form 2 inch round cookies on the prepared sheets.

Bake for 12–15 minutes until a nice golden brown.

Remove from the oven and leave to rest on the cookie sheet for about 5 minutes. Place on a cooling rack.

Serve, eat, and enjoy!

Nutrition:

- Calories: 332 Fat: 13.6g

- Carbs: 48.8g,Dietary Fiber: 2.4g

Protein: 4.9g.

CHAPTER 12:

Desserts

43.   Berries in Crepes

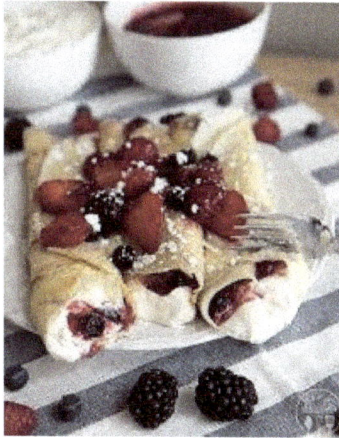

Preparation time: 15 minutes

Cooking time: 20 minutes

Servings: 4

Ingredients:

- 1/2 cup all-purpose flour

- 1/2 cup almond milk

- 2 egg whites, beaten

- 1 tablespoon vegetable oil

- Cooking spray

- 1/2 cup frozen berries (mix of strawberries, raspberries, blueberries), thawed and drained

- 1 tablespoon powdered sugar.

Directions:

In a bowl, mix the flour, almond milk, egg whites, and oil. Spray oil on your pan. Turn the stove to medium heat. Pour 1/4 cup of the flour mixture into the pan. Let the batter spread by moving the pan in a circular motion. Cook until golden. Put the berries on top of the crepe. Let it cook for another 2 minutes before folding the crepe in half. Repeat for the rest of the batter. Sprinkle powdered sugar on top before serving.

Nutrition:

- Calories: 124

- Protein: 5g

- Carbohydrates: 17g

- Fat: 4g

- Cholesterol: 0mg

- Sodium: 41mg

- Potassium: 123mg

- Phosphorus: 55mg

- Calcium: 47mg.

44.   **Baked Egg Custard**

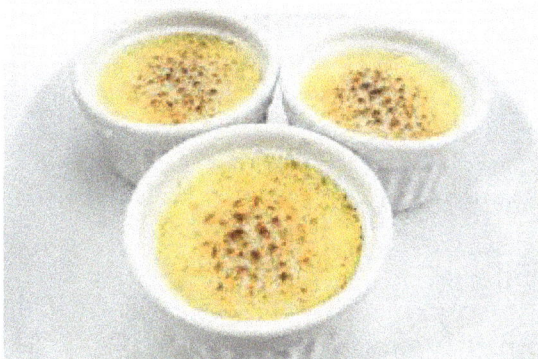

Preparation time: 15 minutes

Cooking time: 30 minutes

Servings: 4
Ingredients:

- 2 medium eggs, at room temperature

- ¼ cup of semi-skimmed milk

- 3 tablespoons of white sugar

- ½ teaspoon of nutmeg

- 1 teaspoon of vanilla extract.

Directions:

Preheat your oven at 375 F/180C

Mix all the ingredients in a mixing bowl and beat with a hand mixer for a few seconds until creamy and uniform.

Pour the mixture into lightly greased muffin tins.

Bake for 25-30 minutes or until the knife you place inside comes out clean.

Nutrition:

- Calories: 96.56

- Carbohydrate: 10.5g

- Protein: 3.5g

- Sodium: 37.75mg

- Potassium: 58.19mg

- Phosphorus: 58.76mg

- Dietary Fiber: 0.06g

- Fat: 2.91 g.

45. Gumdrop Cookies

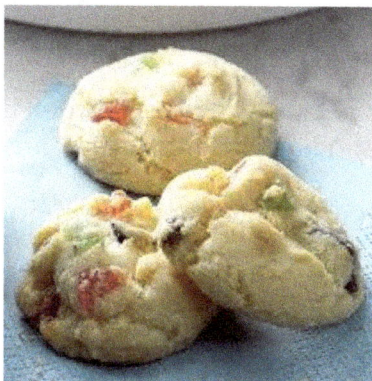

Preparation time: 15 minutes

Cooking time: 12 minutes

Servings: 25
Ingredients:

- ½ cup of spreadable unsalted butter

- 1 medium egg

- 1 cup of brown sugar

- 1 ⅔ cups of all-purpose flour, sifted

- ¼ cup of milk

- 1 teaspoon vanilla

- 1 teaspoon of baking powder

- 15 large gumdrops, chopped finely.

Directions:

Preheat the oven at 400F/195C.

Combine the sugar, butter, and egg until creamy.

Add the milk and vanilla and stir well.

Combine the flour with the baking powder in a different bowl. Incorporate to the sugar, butter mixture, and stir.

Add the gumdrops and place the mixture in the fridge for half an hour.

Drop the dough with tablespoonful into a lightly greased baking or cookie sheet.

Bake for 10-12 minutes or until golden brown.

Nutrition:

- Calories: 102.17

- Carbohydrate: 16.5g

- Protein: 0.86g

- Sodium: 23.42mg

- Potassium: 45mg

- Phosphorus: 32.15mg

- Dietary Fiber: 0.13 g

- Fat: 4g.

46. Pound Cake with Pineapple

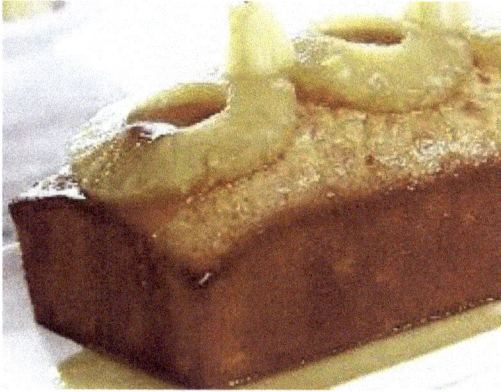

Preparation time: 10 minutes

Cooking time: 50 minutes

Servings: 24
Ingredients:

- 3 cups of all-purpose flour, sifted

- 3 cups of sugar

- 1 ½ cups of butter

- 6 whole eggs and 3 egg whites

- 1 teaspoon of vanilla extract

- 1 10. Ounce can of pineapple chunks, rinsed and crushed (keep juice aside).

For glaze:

- 1 cup of sugar

- 1 stick of unsalted butter or margarine

- Reserved juice from the pineapple.

Directions:

Preheat the oven at 350F/180C.

Beat the sugar and the butter with a hand mixer until creamy and smooth. Slowly add the eggs (one or two every time) and stir well after pouring each egg. Add the vanilla extract, follow up with the flour and stir well. Add the drained and chopped pineapple. Pour the mixture into a greased cake tin and bake for 45-50 minutes. In a small saucepan, combine the sugar with the butter and pineapple juice. Stir every few seconds and bring to boil. Cook until you get a creamy to thick glaze consistency. Pour the glaze over the cake while still hot. Let cook for at least 10 seconds and serve.

Nutrition:

- Calories: 407.4 Carbohydrate: 79g

- Protein: 4.25g Sodium: 118.97mg

- Potassium: 180.32mg

- Phosphorus: 66.37mg

- Dietary Fiber: 2.25 g

- Fat: 16.48g.

47. **Apple Crunch Pie**

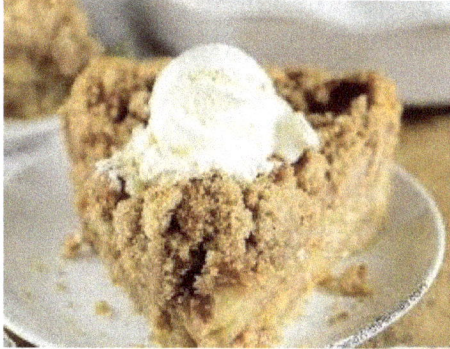

Preparation time: 10 minutes

Cooking time: 35 minutes

Servings: 8
Ingredients:

- 4 large tart apples, peeled, seeded, and sliced

- ½ cup of all-purpose white flour

- ⅓ Cup margarine

- 1 cup of sugar

- ¾ cup of rolled oat flakes

- ½ teaspoon of ground nutmeg.

Directions:

Preheat the oven to 375F/180C.

Place the apples over a lightly greased square pan (around 7 inches).

Mix the rest of the ingredients in a medium bowl with and spread the batter over the apples. Bake for 30-35 minutes or until the top crust has gotten golden brown.

Serve hot.

Nutrition:

- Calories: 261.9

- Carbohydrate: 47.2g

- Protein: 1.5g

- Sodium: 81mg

- Potassium: 123.74mg

- Phosphorus: 35.27mg

- Dietary Fiber: 2.81 g

- Fat: 7.99 g.

48. Spiced Peaches

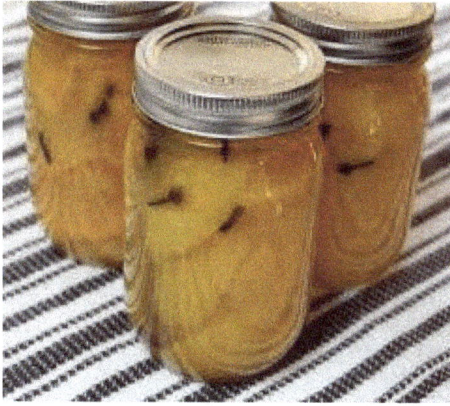

Preparation time: 5 minutes

Cooking time: 10 minutes

Servings: 2
Ingredients:

- 1 cup canned peaches with juices

- ½ teaspoon cornstarch

- 1 teaspoon ground cloves

- 1 teaspoon ground cinnamon

- 1 teaspoon ground nutmeg

- ½ lemon zest

- ½ cup water.

Directions:

Drain peaches.

Combine cinnamon, cornstarch, nutmeg, ground cloves, and lemon zest in a pan on the stove. Heat over medium heat and add peaches. Bring to a boil, reduce the heat and simmer for 10 minutes.

Serve.

Nutrition:

- Calories: 70

- Fat: 0g

- Carb: 14g

- Phosphorus: 23mg

- Potassium: 176mg

- Sodium: 3mg

- Protein: 1g.

49.   Pumpkin Cheesecake Bar

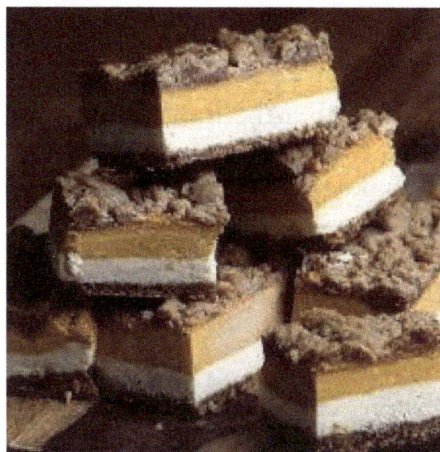

Preparation time: 10 minutes

Cooking time: 50 minutes

Servings: 4
Ingredients:

- 2 ½ tablespoons unsalted butter

- 4 ounces cream cheese

- ½ cup all-purpose white flour

- 3 tablespoons golden brown sugar

- ¼ cup granulated sugar

- ½ cup pureed pumpkin

- 2 egg whites

- 1 teaspoon ground cinnamon

- 1 teaspoon ground nutmeg

- 1 teaspoon vanilla extract.

Directions:

Preheat the oven to 350F. Mix flour and brown sugar in a bowl. Mix in the butter to form 'breadcrumbs. Place ¾ of this mixture in a dish. Bake in the oven for 15 minutes. Remove and cool.

Lightly whisk the egg and fold in the cream cheese, sugar, pumpkin, cinnamon, nutmeg and vanilla until smooth.

Pour this mixture over the oven-baked base and sprinkle with the rest of the breadcrumbs from earlier.

Bake in the oven for 30 to 35 minutes more.

Cool, slice, and serve.

Nutrition:

- Calories: 248

- Fat: 13g

- Carb: 33g

- Phosphorus: 67mg

- Potassium: 96mg

- Sodium: 146mg

- Protein: 4g.

50. Grilled Pineapple

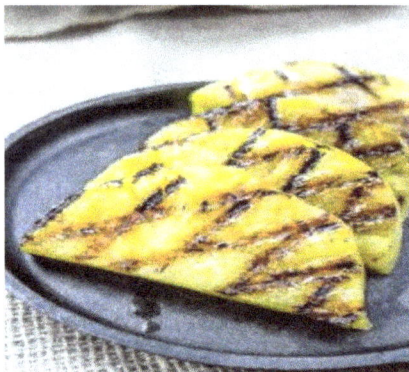

Preparation time: 7 minutes

Cooking time: 5 minutes

Servings: 4

Ingredients:

- 10 oz. fresh pineapple

- ½ teaspoon ground ginger

- 1 tablespoon almond butter, softened.

Directions:

Slice the pineapple into the serving pieces and brush with almond butter. After this, sprinkle every pineapple piece with ground ginger. Preheat the grill to 400F. Grill the pineapple for 2 minutes from each side. The cooked fruit should have a light brown surface on both sides.

Nutrition:

- Calories: 61 Fat: 2.4g Fiber: 1.4g

- Carbs 10.2g Protein: 1.3g

Conclusion

Prevention of diseases that can affect the kidneys starts at the table. Nutrition: plays a fundamental role in ensuring the health of these organs, which perform some essential functions for the body..

The kidneys are organs responsible for the filtration of blood; therefore, they are essential for human life.

The diet plays a key role in maintaining kidney health; in fact, the scraps of all the previously digested-absorbed-metabolized nutritional molecules are filtered by the circulatory stream thanks to the kidney, then collected in the bladder and expelled with urine through urination.

CPSIA information can be obtained
at www.ICGtesting.com
Printed in the USA
BVHW012219230321
603253BV00004B/68

9 781914 421211